DIAGNOSTIC AND MASTERY TESTS TO ACCOMPANY

Foundations First

SENTENCES AND PARAGRAPHS

Bedford/St. Martin's

Boston ■ New York

Preface

Diagnostic and Mastery Tests to Accompany FOUNDATIONS FIRST: SENTENCES AND PARAGRAPHS includes the following diagnostic and review materials:

- The Sentence Skills Diagnostic Test comprises fifty items and covers the grammar, punctuation, and mechanics topics in Units 2–5 of *Foundations First*. (This diagnostic test is also available online at the Exercise Central Web site, which can be reached via <http://www.bedfordstmartins.com/foundationsfirst>.)

- Forty-two review exercise sets test students' mastery of the material in Units 2–5 of *Foundations First*. Two tests are included for each chapter, challenging students to complete both discrete item sets and connected-discourse editing exercises.

Answers to the diagnostic and mastery tests are provided in the Answers section at the end of the booklet. The diagnostic key includes cross-references to relevant chapters in *Foundations First* and to relevant exercises in the Exercise Central collection.

Also available with *Foundations First* are an exercise booklet, *Supplemental Exercises to Accompany* FOUNDATIONS FIRST, and a 700-item electronic exercise bank at the Bedford/St. Martin's online exercise site, Exercise Central, which can be accessed at <http://www.bedfordstmartins.com/foundationsfirst>. If you would like more information about these exercise materials or about the complete supplements package for *Foundations First*, please contact your local Bedford/St. Martin's sales rep or e-mail <sales _support@bfwpub.com>.

Manufactured in the United States of America.

6 5   4   3   2
f   e   d   c   b   a

For information, write: Bedford/St. Martin's, 75 Arlington Street, Boston, MA 02116   (617-399-4000)

ISBN: 0-312-39425-X

Contents

Understanding Basic Grammar

Understanding Punctuation, Mechanics, and Spelling

Sentence Skills Diagnostic Test

Many of the following numbered items are not complete sentences or contain grammatical errors or other writing problems. From the choices following each item, select the best sentence and circle the corresponding letter. If you think the original item is the best option, select "NO CHANGE."

1. The Midwestern speech pattern of most news anchors with no accent.
    a. The Midwestern speech pattern of most news anchors does not sound like an accent to many Americans.
    b. Hearing the Midwestern speech pattern of most news anchors without an accent.
    c. NO CHANGE

2. The largest one of the guard dogs pose no threat to anyone.
    a. The largest one of the guard dogs poses no threat to anyone.
    b. The largest one of the guard dog poses no threat to anyone.
    c. NO CHANGE

3. The owl hooted eerily as we hide in the woods behind the house.
    a. The owl hooted eerily as we hid in the woods behind the house.
    b. The owl hoots eerily as we hid in the woods behind the house.
    c. NO CHANGE

4. Mildred annoyed the cleaning staff leaving muddy footprints.
    a. Leaving muddy footprints, Mildred annoyed the cleaning staff.
    b. Mildred annoyed, leaving muddy footprints, the cleaning staff.
    c. NO CHANGE

5. The doctor told me to quit smoking.
    a. The doctor telling me to quit smoking.
    b. The doctor told me to quit smoking.
    c. NO CHANGE

6. Nancy and I agreed to walk four miles before work each day, but she is more willing to exercise than I.
    a. Nancy and me agreed to walk four miles before work each day, but she is more willing to exercise than me.
    b. Nancy and I agreed to walk four miles before work each day, but she is more willing to exercise than me.
    c. NO CHANGE

7. I told the artist that the sculpture was the unusualest thing I had ever seen.
    a. I told the artist that the sculpture was the most unusual thing I had ever seen.
    b. I told the artist that the sculpture was the most unusualest thing I had ever seen.
    c. NO CHANGE

1

8. People with problems seek out Geert because he gives excellent advices.
    a. People with problems seek out Geert because he gives excellent advice.
    b. People with problems seek out Geert because he gives an excellent advice.
    c. NO CHANGE

9. Idaho, a state with many conservative and right-wing inhabitants also has a huge number of organic farms.
    a. Idaho, a state with many conservative and right-wing inhabitants, also has a huge number of organic farms.
    b. Idaho a state with many conservative and right-wing inhabitants also has a huge number of organic farms.
    c. NO CHANGE

10. Isadora Duncan should'nt have worn a long scarf in a convertible.
    a. Isadora Duncan shouldn't have worn a long scarf in a convertible.
    b. Isadora Duncan shouldnt have worn a long scarf in a convertible.
    c. NO CHANGE

11. She wants to be left alone more than being recognized in public.
    a. She would prefer being left alone more than to be recognized in public.
    b. She likes to be left alone more than to be recognized in public.
    c. NO CHANGE

12. Her parents allowed her band to practice in their garage, they refused to let the musicians turn their amplifiers all the way up.
    a. Her parents allowed her band to practice in their garage, but they refused to let the musicians turn their amplifiers all the way up.
    b. Her parents allowed her band to practice in their garage, however, they refused to let the musicians turn their amplifiers all the way up.
    c. NO CHANGE

13. Is supposed to rain tomorrow and ruin our plans.
    a. Is supposed to rain tomorrow and to ruin our plans.
    b. It is supposed to rain tomorrow and ruin our plans.
    c. NO CHANGE

14. A doctor must abide by the Hippocratic Oath from medical school until retirement.
    a. A doctor must abide by the Hippocratic Oath from their student days until retirement.
    b. A doctor must abide by the Hippocratic Oath from their student days until they retire.
    c. NO CHANGE

15. There is many reasons for instructors to penalize late papers.
    a. There are many reasons for instructors to penalize late papers.
    b. There is a lot of reasons for instructors to penalize late papers.
    c. NO CHANGE

16. The son of a tremendously wealthy mine owner, William Randolph Hearst grew up believing that he could buy anything he wanted.
    a. The son of a tremendously wealthy mine owner William Randolph Hearst grew up believing that he could buy anything he wanted.
    b. The son of a tremendously wealthy mine owner William Randolph Hearst, grew up believing that he could buy anything he wanted.
    c. NO CHANGE

17. In 1965, when integration was hotly debated in the United States, Flannery O'Connor published her story "Everything That Rises Must Converge".
    a. In 1965, when integration was hotly debated in the United States, Flannery O'Connor published her story *Everything That Rises Must Converge*.
    b. In 1965, when integration was hotly debated in the United States, Flannery O'Connor published her story "Everything That Rises Must Converge."
    c. NO CHANGE

18. My history assignment is to read *The Devil in Massachusetts*, watch *The Crucible*, and I have to write a paper about the Salem witch trials.
    a. My history assignment is to read *The Devil in Massachusetts*, to watch *The Crucible*, followed by my writing a paper about the Salem witch trials.
    b. My history assignment is to read *The Devil in Massachusetts*, watch *The Crucible*, and write a paper about the Salem witch trials.
    c. NO CHANGE

19. A cold wind was blowing when Marisa arrived to Chicago.
    a. A cold wind was blowing when Marisa arrived at Chicago.
    b. A cold wind was blowing when Marisa arrived in Chicago.
    c. NO CHANGE

20. Its true that our vacation was not as expensive as their's was.
    a. It's true that our vacation was not as expensive as theirs was.
    b. Its true that our vacation was not as expensive as theirs was.
    c. NO CHANGE

21. The congressman has a metal hip he had difficulty passing through the airport security checkpoint.
    a. The congressman has a metal hip, he had difficulty passing through the airport security checkpoint.
    b. The congressman has a metal hip; he had difficulty passing through the airport security checkpoint.
    c. NO CHANGE

22. She joining the cross-country track team at school.
    a. Been running on the cross-country track team at school.
    b. She has joined the cross-country track team at school.
    c. NO CHANGE

23. Firefighters deserve respect, for you have to be brave to enter burning buildings.
    a. Firefighters deserve respect, for they have to be brave to enter burning buildings.
    b. A firefighter deserves respect, for they have to be brave to enter burning buildings.
    c. NO CHANGE

24. I planned to buy a ticket, but I could not raise enough money.
    a. I planned to buy a ticket, but I cannot raise enough money.
    b. I planted to buy a ticket, but I could not raise enough money.
    c. NO CHANGE

25. The state boxing commission refused to give their permission for the fight.
    a. The state boxing commission refused to give its permission for the fight.
    b. The state boxing commission refused to give his or her permission for the fight.
    c. NO CHANGE

26. He did not feel well, but he knew that his new suit looked well.
    a. He did not feel well, but he knew that his new suit looked good.
    b. He did not feel good, but he knew that his new suit looked well.
    c. NO CHANGE

27. Tom and Marge have went to the jazz festival every summer for six years.
    a. Tom and Marge have go to the jazz festival every summer for six years.
    b. Tom and Marge have gone to the jazz festival every summer for six years.
    c. NO CHANGE

28. Greta always knows the correct answer before anyone else.
    a. Greta is always knowing the correct answer before anyone else.
    b. Greta does always knows the correct answer before anyone else.
    c. NO CHANGE

29. Not letting credit card debt pile up in the first place is much easier than finding a way out of it.
    a. Not letting credit card debt pile up in the first place is much easier than to find a way out of it.
    b. Not to let credit card debt pile up in the first place is much easier than finding a way out of it.
    c. NO CHANGE

30. A boat that sails long distances should have a generator.
    a. A boat that sail long distances should have a generator.
    b. Boats that sails long distances should have generators.
    c. NO CHANGE

31. The Arab world, which had excellent libraries in medieval times, was then far ahead of Europe in scientific achievements.
    a. The Arab world which had excellent libraries in medieval times was then far ahead of Europe in scientific achievements.

b. The Arab world, which had excellent libraries in medieval times was then far ahead of Europe in scientific achievements.
c. NO CHANGE

32. "I'm sorry, I said, "But I don't remember meeting you before."
    a. "I'm sorry", I said but I don't remember meeting you before."
    b. "I'm sorry," I said, "but I don't remember meeting you before."
    c. NO CHANGE

33. The president was mired in a scandal; around the country, journalists wondered if anyone cared.
    a. The president was mired in a scandal, around the country, journalists wondered if anyone cared.
    b. The president was mired in a scandal around the country, journalists wondered if anyone cared.
    c. NO CHANGE

34. The new employee asked if I wanted fries with my order.
    a. The new employee asked did I want fries with my order?
    b. The new employee asked, "Did I want fries with my order?"
    c. NO CHANGE

35. Leaping and spinning, the skater whipping past us through the winter air.
    a. With a leap and a spin, the skater whipping past us through the winter air.
    b. Leaping and spinning, the skater went whipping past us through the winter air.
    c. NO CHANGE

36. He chosen her as his partner for every debate that spring.
    a. He chose her as his partner for every debate that spring.
    b. He choosed her as his partner for every debate that spring.
    c. NO CHANGE

37. Either of the boys would have given up their summer vacation to play in the minor leagues.
    a. Either of the boys would have given up his or her summer vacation to play in the minor leagues.
    b. Either of the boys would have given up his summer vacation to play in the minor leagues.
    c. NO CHANGE

38. His job is only way for his family to support itself.
    a. His job is the only way for his family to support itself.
    b. His job is an only way for the family to support itself.
    c. NO CHANGE

39. The work however, must be done quickly, cheaply and well.
    a. The work, however, must be done quickly, cheaply, and well.
    b. The work, however must be done quickly cheaply, and well.
    c. NO CHANGE

40. Someone win the prize money at the end of the contest.
   a. Someone wins the prize money at the end of the contest.
   b. Somebody win the prize money at the end of the contest.
   c. NO CHANGE

41. With their high-pitched barking, some apartment buildings do not allow small dogs.
   a. Some apartment buildings, with their high-pitched barking, do not allow small dogs.
   b. Some apartment buildings do not allow small dogs with their high-pitched barking.
   c. NO CHANGE

42. The chief executive has taken millions of dollars' worth of stock options instead of a raise in pay.
   a. The chief executive has took millions of dollars' worth of stock options instead of a rise in pay.
   b. The chief executive has taked millions of dollars' worth of stock options instead of a raise in pay.
   c. NO CHANGE

43. The babysitter who she was supposed to come at six o'clock never arrived.
   a. The babysitter who was supposed to come at six o'clock she never arrived.
   b. The babysitter who was supposed to come at six o'clock never arrived.
   c. NO CHANGE

44. I don't remember whether Harold or Georg said that he would take the old tires to the dump.
   a. I don't remember whether Harold or Georg said that they would take the old tires to the dump.
   b. I don't remember whether Harold or Georg said that, they would take the old tires to the dump.
   c. NO CHANGE

45. Sixteen clowns jumped out of a little red tin car.
   a. Sixteen clowns jumped out of a red tin little car.
   b. Sixteen clowns jumped out of a tin red little car.
   c. NO CHANGE

46. The more active the child, the more certainer the parents are to feel exhausted all the time.
   a. The activer the child, the certainer the parents are to feel exhausted all the time.
   b. The more active the child, the more certain the parents are to feel exhausted all the time.
   c. NO CHANGE

47. The town's drugstore still has a soda fountain where customers can get a chocolate malt.
   a. The town's drugstore still has a soda fountain where you can get a chocolate malt.

b. The town's drugstore still has a soda fountain where a chocolate malt can be gotten.
c. NO CHANGE

48. Sam or the twins wins the chili-cooking contest every year.
    a. The twins or Sam win the chili-cooking contest every year.
    b. Sam or the twins win the chili-cooking contest every year.
    c. NO CHANGE

49. Wailing loudly, Roberto carried the baby around and around the living room.
    a. Roberto carried the baby, wailing loudly, around and around the living room.
    b. Roberto carried the baby around and around the living room, wailing loudly.
    c. NO CHANGE

50. The college's work-study program pays some students a little money.
    a. The college's work-study program pays some student a little money.
    b. The college's work-study program pays some student a few money.
    c. NO CHANGE

◆ 6.1 Writing Simple Sentences

For each of the following sentences, underline the complete subject once and the complete verb twice. Enclose any prepositional phrases in parentheses. Then label the simple subject (S) and the verb (AV for action verb or LV for linking verb).

1. A caterpillar spun its cocoon on a milkweed stalk beside the road.

2. Our bathroom window is allowing water into the wall above the bathtub.

3. After reading six novels about the British navy, Howard still doesn't know a frigate from a schooner.

4. On the other side of the valley, a tornado flattened several trees two years ago.

5. The F.B.I. agents standing in the doorway were not making a social call.

6. Surely you can understand my objections to the opinions on this Web site.

7. The runt of the litter looked hungry and cold.

8. The campsites on the map of this national forest seem too distant from the highway.

9. Since his birthday party last year, everyone in the dorm has considered him a lunatic.

10. The smallest variety of lizard is about the size of a dime.

11. Threatened with arrest, the shouting protesters outside City Hall collapsed onto the sidewalk.

12. The new administration's candidates for cabinet posts have been almost completely without government experience.

13. The horses at the hitching post outside the saloon waited patiently for their riders' return.

14. In an election year, environmental issues and the economy appear essential to many politicians.

15. The odd-looking bald man and his clever dog are world travelers.

16. The sun lamp turned all of the patrons a hideous orange color.

17. Kathy wore her little sister's wedding dress for the big day.

18. After the stroke, my strong-willed aunt was very fortunate in her recovery.

19. A patent or other government license does not guarantee the effectiveness of vitamins and herbal supplements.

20. At dusk, hundreds of tourists outside the mouth of the cave watched the nightly departure of the bats.

◆ 6.2 Writing Simple Sentences

For each of the following sentences underline the complete subject once and the complete verb twice. Enclose any prepositional phrases in parentheses. Then label the simple subject (S) and the verb (AV for action verb or LV for linking verb).

1. The peanut butter in the cupboard has become stale.

2. One of the children has thrown a sandwich into the wastebasket.

3. After lunch, the youngest girl announced her preference for cheese sandwiches.

4. Privately, all three teachers at the preschool would agree with her.

5. To the children at the preschool, napping does not often come easily.

6. They are excited about the other children and the toys.

7. On the other hand, the adults have always counted on nap time for cleaning up.

8. Jelly-covered fingers leave sticky marks on the walls and furniture.

9. Emily has been spending six hours in day care every day since a month after her birth.

10. Her younger brother and sister will soon be attending the same day care center.

11. Everyone at preschool, including the teachers, sings with gusto during music time.

12. A college degree and current information about early childhood development are not necessary for this type of work.

13. Are the rewards of playing and singing with little boys and girls enough for most people?

14. A job working with infants and toddlers seems too difficult for some adults.

15. In the United States, childcare providers receive low wages and little respect.

16. With so few incentives, some extremely dedicated people go into the field of child care.

17. Unfortunately, some completely unqualified and uninterested people care for young children, too.

18. Other countries make good child care a priority by paying good wages for the service.

19. Shouldn't the welfare of children be important even to Americans without young children of their own?

20. A good start in life can make a big difference for the child, for the parents, and for the rest of society.

◆ 7.1   Writing Compound Sentences

Combine the two sentences in each pair by using one of the coordinating conjunctions listed below. Choose a conjunction that is appropriate for the relationship between the ideas expressed in the two sentences. Be sure to punctuate the sentence correctly.

Coordinating conjunctions: and   but   for   nor   or   so   yet

1. The chicken flapped its wings. It could not fly.

   _____

   _____

2. The stapler did not work properly. He opened it.

   _____

   _____

3. My baby daughter cries frequently. She cannot communicate with us any other way.

   _____

   _____

4. He could not understand Arabic. He could not read the French subtitles.

   _____

   _____

5. You could change the opening paragraph. You could just clarify the thesis statement.

   _____

   _____

6. He went to clean the house on Friday. The owners had forgotten to leave him a key.

   _____

   _____

7. Pakistan has atomic weapons. That fact frightens some people in India.

   _____

   _____

8. Training a dog requires consistency. The whole family should treat the dog the same way.

   _____

   _____

9. The teacher was prepared for the lesson. The students had done their homework.

   _____

   _____

10. Punk rock continues to attract new fans. It has been around for thirty years.

    _____

    _____

Combine the two sentences in each pair by using a semicolon alone or with one of the conjunctive adverbs or transitional expressions listed. Choose a conjunctive adverb or transitional expression that is appropriate for the relationship between the ideas expressed in the two sentences. Be sure to punctuate each new sentence correctly.

Conjunctive adverbs:	besides	consequently	however	still
	instead	nevertheless	therefore	

Transitional expressions:	for example	in fact
	in addition	as a result

11. Most cable television shows attract small audiences. Many of the shows are well acted and well written.

    _____

    _____

12. Carla's suitcase was not on her connecting flight. She arrived with only a toothbrush.

    _____

    _____

13. The enchiladas were delicious. They tasted even better than my mother's.

    _____

    _____

14. Marcus's company went out of business in May. He has managed to pay his rent on time.

    _____

    _____

15. This letter to the editor contains some inaccurate information. Very few local people supported the council members' proposal.

_____

_____

16. Tomas received the highest score on the midterm exam. He was on time for every class session.

_____

_____

17. The public ignored the scandal. Newspapers and television shows discussed nothing else.

_____

_____

18. My credit card bills were breaking my budget. I had to stop using the cards.

_____

_____

19. Every bite caused terrible pain in my tooth. I avoided seeing my dentist.

_____

_____

20. Each year in the Chinese calendar is named for an animal. This is the Year of the Ox.

_____

_____

◆ 7.2 Writing Compound Sentences

The following passages consist of short, choppy sentences. Revise each passage by linking pairs of sentences with a coordinating conjunction or with a semicolon and a conjunctive adverb or transitional expression. The revision should be a smoothly written paragraph that connects ideas clearly and logically. Be sure to punctuate correctly.

a.   (1) Weather forecasters often get to appear on television. (2) The job offers some prestige. (3) Forecasting the weather seems like an attractive position to many Americans. (4) Weather forecasting does not seem so appealing in some other countries. (5) A weatherman in Rio de Janeiro forecast rain on New Year's Eve. (6) Continual rainstorms had dampened many Brazilians' spirits. (7) Many people simply stayed away from the outdoor celebration. (8) The New Year's Eve party was a flop. (9) The predicted rain never arrived. (10) The weatherman was sent to jail for his mistake.

b.   (1) Asthma affects nine million American children. (2) Smog has long been blamed for making the chronic illness worse. (3) Poor air quality actually seems to cause asthma. (4) A study followed children in twelve communities in southern California for ten years. (5) The results were published in a respected medical journal. (6) The children were reasonably healthy to begin with. (7) All participated in athletics. (8) Six of the communities had fairly clean air. (9) The rest had some of the poorest air quality in the United States. (10) The children in smoggy areas were three to four times more likely to develop asthma.

◆ 8.1 Writing Complex Sentences

Combine the two sentences in each pair by using one of the subordinating conjunctions listed. Choose a conjunction that is appropriate for the relationship between the ideas expressed in the two sentences. Be sure to punctuate correctly.

Subordinating conjunctions:

after	before	while	when
because	as	although	since
so that	until		

1. I felt good about my performance on the test. I received only an average grade.

   _____

   _____

2. Rajiv stopped delivery of his newspapers and mail. He went out of town for the weekend.

   _____

   _____

3. The employees were picketing outside the factory. The manager was training replacement workers.

   _____

   _____

4. The fans stood and roared. The pitcher walked a third batter.

   _____

   _____

5. She cleaned houses and offices. She finished her degree and went to law school.

   _____

   _____

6. Andreas has a learning disability. He receives extra time for his examinations.

   _____

   _____

7. Beatrice spent the night watching over her sick son. She was exhausted.

   _____

   _____

8. One small boy watched. The other children played in the schoolyard.

_____

_____

9. I took my car for a tuneup. It will get me safely to my parents' house in Oklahoma.

_____

_____

10. Huey has been living in the suburbs. He has found new pastimes.

_____

_____

Combine the two sentences in each pair by using one of the relative pronouns listed. Choose a pronoun that is appropriate for the relationship between the ideas expressed in the two sentences. Be sure to punctuate each new sentence correctly, paying particular attention to restrictive and nonrestrictive ideas.

   Relative pronouns: who   which   that   whose

11. Ida Lupino acted in many well-known films. She also earned respect as a director.

_____

_____

12. My doctor's husband is an accountant. She keeps her billing information in an old shoebox.

_____

_____

13. The tree hangs over his driveway. It stands on his neighbor's property.

_____

_____

14. This old farm has been in Raul's family for decades. It seldom makes a profit.

_____

_____

15. Children eat a lot of candy. They often get cavities.

_____

_____

16. Internet stock prices had been unrealistically high. They fell quickly.

_____

_____

17. William Wegman's photographs of dogs made him famous. Wegman began taking pictures of his Weimaraner named Man Ray.

_____

_____

18. The letter is on the table. It has no return address.

_____

_____

19. This office has no window. It is the only available one on this floor.

_____

_____

20. The town has a declining population. The centennial celebration for the town took place last year.

_____

_____

◆ 8.2   Writing Complex Sentences

The following passage consists of short, choppy sentences. Revise it by linking pairs of sentences with a subordinating conjunction or a relative pronoun. The revision should be a smoothly written passage that connects ideas clearly and logically. Be sure to punctuate correctly.

(1) Harold Russell was working in a market in Massachusetts. (2) The United States entered World War II. (3) Russell considered himself a failure. (4) He immediately enlisted in the army. (5) Russell trained as a paratrooper. (6) He also learned demolition. (7) Demolition earned him a position as an instructor. (8) The D-Day invasion was taking place. (9) Harold Russell was teaching soldiers in North Carolina. (10) He was holding some TNT. (11) It turned out to have a faulty fuse. (12) The bomb exploded in his hands. (13) They had to be amputated and replaced with steel hooks.

(14) Russell became extremely skilled at using the hooks. (15) He made a training film for other disabled soldiers. (16) The Hollywood director William Wyler saw the film. (17) He cast Russell in the movie *The Best Years of Our Lives*. (18) Harold Russell had never acted in his life. (19) He won the Oscar for best supporting actor in 1946. (20) Russell then retired from acting to work for veterans' causes.

◆ 9.1   Fine-Tuning Your Sentences

Revise the following passage for sentence variety, exact words, and concise language. Vary some sentence openings so that not all sentences begin with the subject; replace general words with specific ones; and eliminate or replace wordy, repetitive language.

(1) Smallpox was still infecting fifty million people a year in the 1950s. (2) The World Health Organization campaigned to vaccinate as many people as possible. (3) This bad disease had disappeared by the 1970s. (4) People around the world were supposedly safe and no longer in danger from smallpox. (5) Vaccination against smallpox stopped as a result.

(6) The smallpox virus was stored in two places, top-security laboratories in Russia and one in the United States. (7) It was supposedly a fact that no one but scientists had access to the virus. (8) They studied the virus and ways to defeat it under secure and sterile conditions. (9) The World Health Organization planned to destroy the remaining virus stocks in 1999 but changed the deadline to 2002. (10) The reason that the virus was to be destroyed was that then smallpox would no longer exist.

(11) Health officials now suspect that terrorists or evildoers could have the smallpox virus. (12) No one in the United States has been vaccinated since 1979, and this poses a threat. (13) The vaccination loses effectiveness after seven to ten years. (14) Threats of bioterrorism have made people feel bad. (15) The existing supply of the vaccine, unfortunately, is small. (16) Recent efforts to produce more vaccine have not yielded large amounts due to the fact that there were problems. (17) A new, more powerful kind of smallpox vaccine is now being developed and tested. (18) This process could take two or more years, however.

(19) The executive board of the World Health Organization recommended in 2002 delaying the destruction of the virus because the virus can help to develop vaccines and cures. (20) The organization wants research to proceed quickly and rapidly. (21) The members will review the smallpox situation again in 2004 or 2005.

◆ 9.2   Fine-Tuning Your Sentences

Revise the following passage for sentence variety, exact words, and concise language. Vary some sentence openings so that not all sentences begin with the subject; replace general words with specific ones; and eliminate or replace wordy, repetitive language. As you revise, make sure that the relationship between ideas is clear and that you punctuate correctly.

(1) The ability to laugh makes us human. (2) This is an idea that people have believed for centuries. (3) Laughter may occur in animals other than human beings, however. (4) Dogs and even rats may be able to laugh, according to some studies.

(5) A researcher named Patricia Simonet recorded the sounds of playing dogs. (6) The dogs appeared to be panting normally and in a typical fashion. (7) Simonet and her students at Sierra Nevada College analyzed the recordings later. (8) They discovered something interesting: the pants covered more sound frequencies than normal panting does. (9) Dogs in aggressive clashes did not pant in the same way. (10) The research team wondered if the unusual panting could be an indication denoting the fact that the dogs were laughing. (11) When the team broadcast recordings of the dog "laughter" for other dogs, the dogs picked up toys and approached the sound, ready to play.

(12) Rats may laugh, too. (13) They chirp when they wrestle playfully with other rats. (14) They also chirp before mating or receiving morphine in laboratory tests. (15) Brian Knutson of the National Institutes of Health recorded these sounds, and a second researcher, Jaak Panksepp of Bowling Green University, has recorded similar things. (16) Panksepp tickles the rats to make them make sounds. (17) He warns others, "You have to know the rat."

(18) This research might sound silly except for the fact that testing animal laughter has a serious purpose. (19) Neuroscientists can trace the way brains process good things through such research. (20) Laughing dogs and rats may someday increase our understanding of how animals, including humans, communicate.

◆ 10.1 Using Parallelism

Edit the following sentences to eliminate faulty parallelism, making any changes you think are needed to create parallel structure. If the sentence is correct as written, write *C* in the blank following it.

1. You can either pay by writing a personal check or you can use cash at this restaurant. _____

2. The band played too loudly and the tempos they played were too slow. _____

3. Some of the veterans walked briskly, some limped along, and there were also some veterans riding on a float. _____

4. Being in good physical condition is more important for overall health than to be thin. _____

5. The food was greasy, salty, and I found it delicious. _____

6. His argument uses faulty logic, the statistics are misleading, and irrelevant examples are used. _____

7. The inaccurate information appeared in the newspaper, on several Web sites, and in a widely circulated e-mail message. _____

8. *Beowulf* is written in Old English, *The Canterbury Tales* in Middle English, and Shakespeare wrote plays using an early form of modern English. _____

9. Grandmother banded her hens with yellow rings and the pullets were banded with red rings. _____

10. The bathroom looked shabby because of the cracked tile, the fact that the floor was rust-stained, and the mildewed grout. _____

11. Phobias can make people afraid of open spaces or they may fear elevators. _____

12. I wanted neither to go back home nor could I bear to stay there. _____

13. The families on television all feature wisecracking children and immature parents. _____

14. February has to be short because it is dreary, cold, and spring is too close.

_____

15. The speech was not only well written but it also was delivered beautifully.

_____

16. The sweet sixteen party of her dreams would feature a boy band, real flowers in crystal vases, and everyone would do ballroom dancing. _____

17. The pictures that accompany the recipes are out of focus, garishly tinted, and anyone would find them unappetizing. _____

18. The dog trainer commanded the collie to heel, sit, and to stay. _____

19. The tune I heard might have come from a Broadway show, or perhaps a Beatles song was the source of it. _____

20. Looking through the microscope, we could see the individual cells in the onion skin and the cilia on the bacteria. _____

◆ 10.2 Using Parallelism

Edit the following passage to eliminate faulty parallelism, making any changes you think are needed to create parallel structure.

(1) For decades, people with low self-esteem were said to be likely to commit crimes, drug abuse was typical, and they often went to jail. (2) Psychologists frequently blamed a decision to plant a bomb or beating a spouse on a lack of self-respect. (3) Based on the results of psychological tests, schoolchildren were identified as either having confidence or they lacked self-esteem. (4) Experts wanted to protect children with low self-confidence from lives of misery and being criminals. (5) Therefore, for the past twenty years, social workers, psychologists, and those in teaching have all been expected to help children develop a sense of self-worth.

(6) But is low self-esteem really such a terrible problem? (7) Everyone has met at least one person who both possesses plenty of self-confidence and who treats other people badly. (8) Since the first self-esteem tests were administered, young people have become ever more likely to get high scores than performing poorly. (9) However, crime rates, illegal drug use, and the problem of behaving cruelly to other people have not improved in that time. (10) Today, while many young people have high self-esteem, they may neither have good social skills nor do they do well in school.

(11) Some psychologists have begun to think that high self-esteem either is not a huge influence on a person's quality of life or that it actually causes problems for some people. (12) One researcher believes that people with low self-esteem not only may not be harmed by it, but they may actually do better in school than more confident students. (13) He says that students with low self-esteem study more and are pushing themselves harder because they fear that they will not succeed. (14) Another psychologist has found that people with high self-esteem are likely to

hurt other people or they might endanger them. (15) Furthermore, according to psychological research, people who are violent or hate others because of their racial differences do not secretly feel bad about themselves. (16) One psychologist suggested that such people would be better off feeling worse about themselves than to feel better.

(17) At any rate, many psychologists now believe that feeling bad about oneself does not cause terrorism, substance abuse, and recklessly disregarding human life. (18) However, building self-esteem and the fight to love oneself are a part of the culture today in the United States. (19) Americans may decide that low self-esteem is not a terrible problem, or to continue to convince themselves that they are good people. (20) Whatever happens, people today are beginning to debate the value of the idea of self-worth.

◆ 11.1 Run-Ons and Comma Splices

Some of the following items contain run-ons or comma splices. Carefully correct the errors, making sure that you clearly indicate the relationship between ideas and that you punctuate correctly. If a sentence is correct as written, put a *C* in the blank following it.

1. The chess-playing computer defeats every student the programmers insist that the machine cannot really think. _____

2. People's pupils get larger when they see something that they like. _____

3. I wanted to wear something else for the photograph, I discovered that my favorite outfit no longer fits. _____

4. The long-distance telephone company claimed that the problem was with the local one, the local telephone company blamed the long-distance one. _____

5. A regular mole check should be part of an annual physical exam any change in a mole should be reported to a doctor immediately. _____

6. Ever since my co-worker was laid off, my boss expects me to do her job in addition to mine. _____

7. The children at the door are collecting for UNICEF, what shall we give them? _____

8. Flying is cheaper than taking the train on most trips, it also takes less time. _____

9. I like compact fluorescent light bulbs because they save energy my mother likes them because they do not get hot. _____

10. Maria had never realized how violent some fairy tales could be, her daughter had a nightmare after hearing the story of Hansel and Gretel. _____

11. No rain had fallen for weeks in the county the local golf course broke the law by watering the grass. _____

12. The toys were antiques that had belonged to Conrad's grandfather, his mother would not let him touch them. _____

13. You should avoid that professor his tests have nothing to do with the readings he assigns for the class. _____

14. My roommate borrowed my sweater before she returned it, she had it cleaned. _____

15. He had not heard the song in years, it brought back a rush of happy childhood memories. _____

16. Jorge floated on his back in the lake he admired the puffy clouds high in the sky above. _____

17. The grammar checker on this computer gives strange advice, I do not usually use it. _____

18. In the poems, Mehitabel is a cat Archy is a cockroach who was a writer in his previous life. _____

19. Jan has not unpacked the boxes in his basement since he moved five years ago, he probably doesn't really need the items in them. _____

20. While the drivers watched the snow falling and worried about the roads, the skiers rubbed their hands with glee. _____

◆ 11.2 Run-Ons and Comma Splices

The following passage contains several run-on sentences and comma splices. Read the passage, and circle the number before each run-on and comma splice. Then correct the errors, making sure that the connection between ideas is clear and that the revised sentences are correctly punctuated.

(1) When Americans planted trees in their cities and towns, they often planted American elms. (2) These trees are tall their branches are long and graceful. (3) Elms look beautiful along a street, the branches on one side form an arch with the branches on the other side. (4) Settlers put rows and rows of elms along roads to form leafy green avenues. (5) The elm was one of the most common trees in the United States, in some towns it was nearly the only type of tree. (6) Almost every American town has an Elm Street that was named for the stately American elm.

(7) Scientists have a name for a landscape with only one type of plant, they call it a monoculture. (8) Monocultures can cause problems they are much more likely to suffer an epidemic of a disease. (9) That is exactly what happened in the case of the American elm, deadly Dutch elm disease arrived from abroad. (10) The trees had no resistance to Dutch elm disease the disease had no natural enemies in the United States. (11) The climate where elms grew in the United States was perfect for Dutch elm disease as well. (12) The disease killed the elm trees across the United States, in the northern part of the country more than half of all the elms died. (13) Dutch elm disease can move through the root system from tree to tree when several elms are planted in a row, so the popularity of American elms made the disease worse. (14) Isolated trees can sometimes be saved however, that is an expensive and difficult job. (15) Tree experts find it nearly impossible to save large numbers of elms, instead, they can only look for replacements for the dying trees.

(16) American towns today are more likely than in the past to have different kinds of trees and shrubs, monocultures are not as favored now. (17) One reason

for this change was the total devastation caused by Dutch elm disease no one wanted that to happen again. (18) The most susceptible elm trees have already died, this does not mean that tree diseases from abroad no longer concern Americans. (19) Dogwoods, oaks, cedars, and redwoods are suffering now from diseases that were unknown in the United States a few decades ago. (20) Scientists wonder how American trees will respond to such threats, everyone hopes that no other native species will be hurt as badly as the American elms have been.

◆ 12.1 Sentence Fragments

The following passage contains several sentence fragments. Read the passage, and circle the number before each fragment. Then correct each fragment by adding the words necessary to complete it or by attaching it to a nearby sentence that completes the idea.

(1) Michel Nostradame was an astrologer. (2) Who lived in the sixteenth century. (3) Known today as Nostradamus, he wrote four-line poems called quatrains. (4) A book of these poems published in 1555. (5) With the title *Centuries*. (6) These poems were supposed to be prophecies. (7) Of events that would happen someday. (8) The language of the poems was very obscure. (9) Nevertheless, some people believed that the poems were accurate predictions. (10) And hailed Nostradamus as a man who could see the future.

(11) Translations of Nostradamus's poems still sell many copies each year. (12) As new generations hear about the supposed psychic gifts of the sixteenth-century Frenchman. (13) Skeptical readers notice. (14) That the translations often make the quatrains more specific. (15) To make the predictions clear after the fact. (16) Some translators change words to add references to people such as Hitler. (17) That do not appear in the original French. (18) The poems of Nostradamus, carefully translated, are cryptic. (19) They can interpreted to mean almost anything. (20) Psychics today make cryptic predictions that can be claimed to reveal foreknowledge later. (21) Which, as the Nostradamus "prophecies" demonstrates, is a very old trick.

◆ 12.2 Sentence Fragments

The following passage contains several sentence fragments. Read the passage, and circle the number before each fragment. Then correct each fragment by adding the words necessary to complete it or by attaching it to a nearby sentence that completes the idea.

(1) According to linguistic experts. (2) Yiddish began in the tenth century, when Jews from northern France settled in towns on the Rhine. (3) They began to speak the local German dialect. (4) Because many medieval Jews did not want to use their sacred language, Hebrew, at home. (5) However, they wrote the German dialect using Hebrew characters. (6) Avoiding the Roman alphabet because they associated it with Latin. (7) The language that reminded them of Christian persecution. (8) Thus, Yiddish became a language of Jewish households and markets in central Europe.

(9) Laws in Europe in the twelfth and thirteenth centuries prevented Jews from living near Christians. (10) Leading to the creation of Jewish ghettos. (11) The segregation of Jews and Christians created language differences between German and Yiddish. (12) Although Yiddish is officially categorized as Judeo-German. (13) It has somewhat different spelling and grammar from German. (14) Yiddish was the most-used language among European Jews until World War II. (15) When many Yiddish speakers were killed in the Holocaust.

(16) With the arrival of many Jews in the United States between the late 1800s and the 1940s. (17) Yiddish continued to grow. (18) By adding English words. (19) English, which has borrowed from languages all over the world. (20) Took words, phrases, and other linguistic devices from Yiddish, so both languages were broadened by the exchange.

◆ 13.1 Subject-Verb Agreement

For each of the following sentences, decide whether the subject is singular or plural. Then circle the correct present tense verb.

1. Everyone on the team (has/have) to agree to play by the rules.

2. There (is/are) no other children on this block.

3. Her quiet manner and kind voice (attracts/attract) stray dogs and cats to her.

4. One of the boys (wants/want) an ice cream cone.

5. She and her husband (expects/expect) to retire to Arizona next year.

6. Nelson or the Ortega sisters (is/are) hosting the block party.

7. The water in the local rivers and streams (looks/look) clean enough to drink.

8. From all over the world (comes/come) the reports on the news.

9. Most people in this region (does/do) not understand Cantonese.

10. Someone who works here (keeps/keep) drinking the juice I put in the office refrigerator.

11. The dogs or the cat (has/have) knocked over the kitchen wastebasket again.

12. The roller coasters that you can ride in the amusement park (is/are) old and wooden.

13. (Is/Are) this bicycle for sale?

14. The cake and cookies that you baked (does/do) not tempt me after that big dinner.

15. How much time (does/do) a trip like this usually take?

16. The veterinarians at the wildlife park (has/have) fascinating and sometimes dangerous jobs.

17. Either a taxi or a bus (takes/take) about twenty minutes to get to the bridge from here.

18. The woman who returned my wallet with all of the cash and credit cards (deserves/deserve) a reward.

19. Anyone scanning the bulletin boards at the student housing office (is/are) probably looking for an apartment.

20. The new printer, ink cartridge, and paper (has/have) to be delivered by Monday morning.

◆ 13.2 Subject-Verb Agreement

The following passage contains several errors in subject-verb agreement. Decide whether each of the underlined verbs agrees with its subject. If it does not, cross it out and write the correct form in the space above. If it does, write *C* above the verb.

(1) Bears in the wilderness <u>does</u> not like surprises. (2) A human or animal that suddenly appears <u>is</u> threatening to a bear. (3) When threatened, grizzly bears and black bears <u>charges</u> at the frightening creature. (4) Naturally, no one <u>want</u> to be the person on the receiving end of such a charge. (5) Some bears <u>have</u> six-inch claws, and a grizzly at maturity <u>weigh</u> six hundred pounds or more. (6) The walking gait of bears <u>appear</u> lumbering and slow, but a charging bear <u>run</u> faster than a horse.

(7) Hikers often <u>wears</u> bells in bear country. (8) The theory behind this practice <u>is</u> that bears will run away from the unfamiliar sound. (9) In such cases, the hikers and the bears <u>does</u> not meet, and tragedies <u>is</u> prevented. (10) However, not everyone <u>are</u> convinced of the value of bear bells. (11) There <u>has</u> been cases of bears that learn to seek out hikers because hikers <u>are</u> usually carrying food. (12) For such bears, the ringing of the bells <u>sound</u> like a call for lunch.

(13) Every hiker, therefore, <u>need</u> to know what to do in case a bear <u>do</u> charge. (14) Mace and pepper spray sometimes <u>stops</u> a bear from attacking. (15) According to experts, the best things to do <u>are</u> to drop to the ground, making the body as small and unthreatening as possible, and to go limp if the bear <u>bites</u>. (16) Of course, if this information <u>frighten</u> people away from hiking in the bear country, then they will also probably be protected from bear attacks.

◆ 14.1 Illogical Shifts

Edit the following sentences to eliminate illogical shifts in tense, person, and voice. If any sentences are correct as written, write *C* in the blank.

1. My father loved this hat, so it has always been treasured by me. _____

2. The rainstorm passed, and by morning a gorgeous sunrise appears over the mountain. _____

3. Many people like the convenience of online shopping, but you have to pay shipping charges. _____

4. The van behind me was dangerously close to my car, and the driver made me nervous. _____

5. Most people watch a lot of television, but few of them wanted to admit it. _____

6. The little girls wanted pink ballerina tutus, but those dresses were not liked by their mother. _____

7. The musicians played klezmer music, and everyone danced joyfully. _____

8. Sally did not get a part in the play, but she will audition again next year. _____

9. We rowed out into the lake and baited our hooks, and in an instant, a big fish strikes. _____

10. To get a good grade, students should always prepare for exams, and you must keep up with the coursework. _____

11. Before people drink the water, you should boil it for twenty minutes. _____

12. She is allergic to shellfish, so the shrimp was not eaten by her. _____

13. My grandfather told me to expect a surprise in the mail, and then a fruitcake arrives. _____

14. The coffee had to be made by the office staff, and the workers clearly resented the task. _____

15. Your account does not get many messages, but at least you don't get any junk e-mail. _____

16. Howard is so old-fashioned that he owns a record player. _____

17. The newspapers were taken to the recycling center by local youth groups, and the kids also collected cans and glass bottles. _____

18. If someone wants change in the political system, you have to vote. _____

19. I was just about to discover the meaning of life, and then I wake up. _____

20. Fawzia told her that you could get organic vegetables at the supermarket. _____

◆ 14.2 Illogical Shifts

The following passage contains a number of sentences with illogical shifts in tense, person, and voice. Read the passage, and circle the number before each sentence containing an illogical shift. Then revise these sentences to eliminate the illogical shifts. Note that some sentences may contain more than one type of illogical shift.

(1) My friend Angel told me that you could sign up for a bicycle ride across the state. (2) I had always enjoyed cycling, although such a long distance had never been ridden by me. (3) Angel also mentioned that you could get sponsors to agree to pay a certain amount to a charity for every mile cycled. (4) I decided that I want to raise money for a good cause. (5) I agreed to join the bicycle ride, and I immediately begin training. (6) I wanted to be in good shape for the ride, so I tried to get fit through hard work and practice.

(7) For several weeks, I biked twenty or thirty miles each day. (8) By late spring, when the statewide ride was scheduled to begin, I feel ready to go. (9) Sponsors had been found by me to contribute to the charity, and all I had to do now was pedal five hundred miles. (10) Angel had planned to ride, too, but he injures his knee in March. (11) I asked his sponsors if they would sponsor me instead, and most agreed. (12) With the potential to earn so much for a good cause, I suddenly realize how important it was for me to complete the ride. (13) Angel told me that you shouldn't think about things like that before a long, strenuous trip.

(14) We set out on our bikes in May, riding from west to east so that you would not be facing into the wind. (15) The western half of the state has higher hills and elevations, so we could also make better time by traveling east. (16) You wanted to do the hardest part of the trip at the beginning, when we were fresh. (17) On the first day, we were passed by fast-moving trucks, and the weather was rainy and miserable. (18) However, I never really thought about quitting because I couldn't have faced the sponsors and the people at the charity if I had quit.

(19) To my surprise, I soon found that I am one of the strongest and fastest cyclists in the group. (20) The five-hundred-mile trip was completed by me a day ahead of schedule, and the charity received a large contribution.

◆ 15.1 Dangling and Misplaced Modifiers

Rewrite the following sentences, which contain dangling and misplaced modifiers, so that each modifier refers to a word or word group it can logically modify.

1. Sweating in the humid sunshine, the tractors moved back and forth across the field.

2. The beaver smacked the water with its broad tail certain of danger.

3. Exhausted after the long drive, our car pulled into the driveway at last.

4. Handmade by my niece, water kept dripping out of the vase.

5. That book kept me awake far into the night that I borrowed from you.

6. A reflecting pool surrounded the temple filled with carp.

7. With nowhere else to turn, the bus station seemed to be her only option.

8. Pretending to smile, the stage was covered with dancing contestants.

9. Turning suddenly cold, snow began to fall.

10. She used paste to put the flowers in the book made of flour and water.

11. Snarling defiantly, the letter carrier tiptoed around the dog.

12. Aching from the long hike, a hole in my sock left me with a huge blister.

13. Taping the bow on top, the package looked perfect.

14. Stuck in the ditch, the mobile phone had never been more useful.

15. The dead tree attracted a squirrel family with a hole in it.

16. Preserved in amber, we discovered an ancient type of beetle.

17. Gothic novels thrill many readers featuring old castles and mysterious strangers.

18. Hundreds of feet over our heads, we gasped as the blimp floated past.

19. I accidentally sent an e-mail to the whole class intended for you alone.

20. Stunned by the revelation, throughout the banquet hall no sound was heard.

◆ 15.2 Dangling and Misplaced Modifiers

The following passage contains some dangling and misplaced modifiers. Read the passage, and circle the number before each sentence containing a dangling or misplaced modifier. Then revise these sentences to eliminate the errors.

(1) An abandoned house attracted three neighborhood children filled with cobwebs and mysterious rooms. (2) Creeping in through the broken window by the porch, nothing had been disturbed for decades. (3) A calendar said that the date was October 1977 on the wall. (4) Sam, Dana, and Eduardo were surprised to find the cupboards filled with boxes and cans looking first in the kitchen. (5) With an ancient yellow label, Eduardo picked up a can of beans. (6) Scuttling across the floor, the children saw that mice had made the house their own. (7) Boxes of cereal with contents that had long ago been eaten by rodents remained on the shelves.

(8) Inching up the steps, the creaks and groans sounded human. (9) The house seemed to be speaking to the children that had been empty for so long. (10) The furnishings reminded them, covered with a thick layer of dust, of things they had seen at their grandparents' houses. (11) Sam wanted to look in the attic, the oldest of the three. (12) Climbing up the ladder to the top of the house, treasures were discovered. (13) Old clothes spilled out of a battered suitcase from the disco era. (14) Dana put on a glittery shirt with sequins that spelled out "Boogie." (15) With four-inch wooden heels, Eduardo tried a pair of platform shoes.

(16) Returning to the house a week later, a portable CD player was brought along. (17) Sam, Dana, and Eduardo opened the suitcase unable to stop giggling. (18) Borrowed from his mother's collection, Sam played a copy of *ABBA's Greatest Hits*. (19) The three danced through the attic adorned with shoes, hats, giant sunglasses, and yards of polyester. (20) Echoing with laughter, the old house seemed to welcome the children's lively presence.

◆ 16.1 Verbs: Past Tense

In the following sentences, fill in the correct past tense form of each verb in parentheses.

(1) Ann Bancroft _____ (decide) to become a polar explorer after reading a book about a famous expedition to Antarctica. (2) Her dream came true when she _____ (cross) the ice at both the North and South Poles. (3) She also _____ (ski) across Antarctica. (4) She and another explorer _____ (cover) this frozen continent in 100 days. (5) They _____ (pull) sleds that had 250 pounds of supplies on them. She is truly a hero!

For each blank in the paragraph below, fill in the past tense form of the appropriate verb from the following list. Use the verb that makes the most sense in context.

> save   search   scorch   arrive   appear   work   walk   honor
>
> mail   award   collapse   burn   contribute   help   brush

When Apollo, a German shepherd, (6) _____ at the Westminster Dog Show, he was not the usual prize-winning dog. This famous dog show usually (7) _____ ribbons to the best-looking dogs. Instead, in February 2002, they (8) _____ Apollo and other search and rescue dogs who (9) _____ people's lives. After the disasters of September 11, 2001, these dogs (10) _____ for people trapped in the wreckage of the World Trade Center in New York City. When the towers (11) _____, many people couldn't get out. Apollo and other dogs (12) _____ the human rescuers find survivors. Apollo first (13) _____ at the World Trade Center only 15 minutes after the towers fell down. Fire (14) _____ all around him. His handler (15) _____ the burning embers off the dog, and they both (16) _____ many hours that day. The dogs (17)_____ on smoldering wreckage and (18) _____ their paws. Dog-lovers all over the country (19) _____ packages of dog booties to New York to protect the dogs' feet. In addition to honoring the dogs and their handlers, the Westminster Dog Show and other sponsors (20) _____ $275,000 to a search and rescue dog organization.

◆ 16.2 Verbs: Past Tense

In the following sentences, fill in the correct past tense form of each verb in parentheses.

1. Black History Month _____ (begin) as Negro History Week.

2. Dr. Carter Woodson, an African American educator, _____ (start) the event in 1926.

3. Dr. Woodson _____ (see) the need for the achievements of African Americans to be recognized.

4. He _____ (do) many years of research on the subject.

5. His publishing company, Associated Publishers, _____ (publish) his book, *The Negro in Our History.*

6. His book _____ (sell) well as a textbook in high schools and colleges.

7. To popularize Negro History Week, Dr. Woodson _____ (send) information to people all over the world.

8. He _____ (give) lectures on the subject in schools and to community gatherings.

9. After Dr. Woodson's death, the Association of Afro-American Life and History _____ (take) over the job of promoting Negro History Week.

10. Because of the work of this organization, Negro History Week _____ (become) Black History Month in 1976.

11. Carter Godwin Woodson _____ (grow) up in a very poor family.

12. He _____ (be) one of nine children born to parents who had been enslaved.

13. Instead of going to school, he _____ (work) in the coal mines of Virginia as a young boy.

14. When he _____ (reach) the age of 20, he was finally able to attend high school.

15. The brilliant student _____ (graduate) from high school after one and a half years.

16. He then _____ (study) at Berea College in Kentucky.

17. Later, he _____ (teach) at his old high school and was appointed principal.

18. Carter Woodson _____ (take) further college courses and earned his master's degree in 1908 and a Ph.D. from Harvard University in 1912.

19. He _____ (have) a distinguished career which included supervising schools in the Philippines.

20. Dr. Woodson _____ (found) the *Journal of Negro History* and was its editor for 40 years.

◆ 17.1 Verbs: Past Participles

In the following sentences, fill in the correct past participle form of the verbs in parentheses.

1. We should have _____ (know) that the key would be _____ (hide) under the doormat.

2. The cook had_____ (break) the eggs into a bowl, and then he had _____ (beat) them lightly with a fork.

3. He had _____ (sleep) soundly and then had _____ (awake) at the first light of morning.

4. Jesse had _____ (throw) the Frisbee to his dog, but another, faster dog has _____ (catch) it in mid-air.

5. Wendy had _____ (write) an angry letter to her friend, but then she had _____ (think) about it and had _____ (tear) it up.

6. Have you _____ (speak) to Roscoe on the telephone or have you _____ (see) him in person?

7. At the last party, everyone had _____ (wear) casual clothes, so I decided that I could wear jeans to the party tonight.

8. The deer have _____ (eat) all the vegetables that we had _____ (grow) so carefully in our garden.

9. When the coach blew her whistle, each of the swimmers had _____ (dive) into the pool and had _____ (swim) as fast as he or she could.

10. A few days after he has been _____ (pay), Spencer usually has already _____ (spend) most of the money.

In the following sentences, fill in the tense of the verb in parentheses that makes the most sense in context. You should use either the present perfect tense or the past perfect tense.

11. The witness for the defense _____ _____ (swear) that the defendant is not guilty of this crime.

12. Melinda proved to be an excellent teacher, even though she _____ never _____ (teach) before this year.

13. The pot on the stove _____ _____ (boil) over before I could turn the heat down.

14. The child admitted, reluctantly, that he _____ _____ (feel) jealous of his baby sister from time to time.

15. By the time baseball camp was over, Jack _____ _____ (raise) his batting average significantly.

16. We realized that we _____ _____ (leave) the apartment door unlocked all day!

17. Since I have been taking the bus instead of driving to work, I _____ _____ (meet) some interesting people.

18. Janice _____ _____ (write) songs since she was 13 years old and still writes them.

19. Before their guests arrived, the young couple _____ _____ (spend) hours cleaning their apartment.

20. Because the cold weather _____ _____ (freeze) the locks on the car doors, we had to use a special spray to unfreeze them.

◆ 17.2 Verbs: Past Participles

The following paragraph contains several errors in the use of past participles and the perfect tenses. Decide whether each of the underlined verbs or participles is in the correct form. If it is incorrect, cross it out and write the correct form in the space above. If it is correct, write *C* above the verb.

(1) Electric lights, <u>invented</u> in 1878, <u>have changed</u> human life profoundly.

(2) Although gas lamps <u>had light</u> streets, homes, and factories for decades, electric light was much more powerful. (3) An Englishman, Joseph Swan, <u>had</u> first <u>patent</u> an electric lamp in 1878, followed by Thomas Edison, who <u>improved</u> it, in 1879.

(4) After fighting over who <u>had</u> really <u>invented</u> the electric light, the two inventors finally <u>join</u> together to start an electric company. (5) Even though people <u>been</u> fascinated by this new wonder, relatively few <u>had ordered</u> electric service. (6) It <u>had took</u> until around 1910 for the invention to become popular.

(7) Ever since, people <u>have relyed</u> on electric light to extend their day. (8) In fact, electric light <u>has eliminated</u> the night for those who wish to ignore it. (9) It <u>has</u> also <u>make</u> the world a safer and more comfortable place. (10) However, some people <u>have wonder</u> if we <u>have overused</u> electric lighting. (11) These advocates of the night claim that we <u>have went</u> against our natural need for darkness.

(12) Electric lights <u>have keeped</u> most of us from being able to see the stars at night.

(13) They <u>have</u> also <u>harmed</u> some plants and animals and <u>use</u> up natural resources.

(14) A "dark sky" movement <u>has emerge</u> and is urging people to turn off unneeded lights at night. (15) Perhaps humans, as well as animals and plants, <u>need</u> a rest from artificial brightness.

◆ 18.1 Nouns

In the sentences that follow, circle the correct form of the noun in each of the underlined pairs.

1. Love is good for your heart, claim <u>Cardiologists/cardiologists</u>, doctors who treat heart disease.

2. The World Heart <u>Federation/federation</u> in 2002 announced that "being in love and being loved helps to keep us healthy and is particularly good for our hearts."

3. This <u>organization/Organization</u>, which is based in <u>Geneva, Switzerland/geneva, switzerland</u> tries to prevent heart disease.

4. A <u>spokesman/spokesmen</u> for this group said that medical research shows that love reduces stress, <u>Depression/depression</u>, and anxiety.

5. These unpleasant <u>emotion/emotions</u> increase a <u>person's/persons'</u> chance of having heart trouble.

6. This news should encourage <u>husbands-to-be/husband-to-bes</u> and <u>wife-to-bes/wives-to-be</u>.

7. "A healthy lifestyle is also necessary in keeping your heart healthy," warns <u>professor/Professor</u> Philip <u>Poole-Wilson/Poole-wilson</u> of <u>Imperial College/Imperial college</u> in London.

8. Our hearts will benefit when we eat <u>dishs/dishes</u> low in saturated fat and exercise instead of being "couch <u>potatos/potatoes</u>."

9. But <u>scientists/scientistes</u> believe that feelings of love are also a big help.

10. There are more and more <u>proofs/proves</u> to back up these <u>believes/beliefs</u>.

11. One <u>studies/study</u> focused on 1,400 <u>mens/men</u> and <u>womens/women</u> with <u>Coronary/coronary</u> artery disease, which often leads to heart attacks.

12. <u>Half/Halve</u> of the <u>patients/patientes</u> who were not married and had no close relationship in their <u>lifes/lives</u> had died at the end of five years.

13. Only 15 percent of the <u>participant/participants</u> who were married or in a close <u>relationship/relationships</u> died of their heart disease.

14. Even a close relationship with a pet can help adults and <u>children/childrens</u> stay healthy.

15. Petting dogs, cats, rabbits, and <u>ponys/ponies</u> can lower blood pressure significantly and contribute to a healthy heart.

16. In one program at a <u>zoo/Zoo</u>, kids who have trouble making <u>friend/friends</u> learned how to get along with others by playing with friendly animals.

17. The youngsters learned to understand and respect the <u>wishs/wishes</u> of the animals.

18. <u>This/These</u> lessons will help them improve their chances of having good relationships with <u>people/peoples</u>.

◆ 18.2 Nouns

In the following paragraph, there are errors in regular and irregular plural noun forms. Decide whether each of the underlined nouns is in the correct form. If it is incorrect, cross it out and write the correct form in the space above. If it is correct, write *C* above the noun.

(1) In recent years, many <u>person</u> have become more concerned about the welfare of animals. (2) Animal <u>advocates</u> are trying to protect both domesticated and wild <u>populationes</u>. (3) One result is that fewer <u>monkies</u>, apes, dogs, and cats are used in laboratory research. (4) Watchdog <u>groupes</u> want to keep all laboratory animals, including <u>mouses</u> and <u>rats,</u> from unnecessary suffering. (5) They argue that much research can be done using computer <u>modeles</u>. (6) Some even say that research should be done on human <u>volunteers</u> because animal anatomy is not the same as that of humans.

(7) Although hunting has also been criticized, hunters argue that they are "harvesting" surplus <u>deers</u> or <u>elks</u> who would otherwise die of starvation. (8) <u>Critices</u> say that the healthiest animals are killed by hunters, while starvation would take the weakest ones. (9) Environmentalists work to protect endangered <u>species</u>. (10) <u>Wolfs</u> have been introduced once again into Yellowstone National Park. (11) <u>Grizzlys</u> in the West are protected against hunting. (12) Laws help ensure the survival of <u>whales,</u> <u>dolphines,</u> and other sea <u>mammales</u>. (13) Human <u>friends</u> of sea cows or manatees instruct <u>fishermens</u> and boaters on how to avoid harming these gentle creatures. (14) There are limits on catching certain kinds of <u>fishs</u>. (15) The flyways of migrating <u>gooses</u> and other birds are protected. (16) Bird <u>enthusiasts</u> support <u>sanctuaryes</u> and urge us to "shoot" birds only with our <u>cameras</u>. (17) Thanks to all these <u>efforts</u>, the relationship between people and animals is improving.

◆ 19.1 Pronouns

In the sentences that follow, circle the correct pronoun in each of the underlined pairs.

1. My best friend and <u>me/I</u> look so much alike that people think we are sisters.

2. You can order a free appetizer or a free desert, but <u>they/it</u> must cost less than five dollars on the menu.

3. <u>Him/He</u> and his girlfriend have been going steady for two years.

4. Everyone is required to have <u>his or her/their</u> parents complete the financial aid application.

5. The coach congratulated the team on <u>its/their</u> surprise victory in the finals against great odds.

6. Celebrities always seem so sure of <u>theirselves/themselves</u>, but I wonder if they really are.

7. <u>Him and her/He and she</u> are engaged to be married next June.

8. Do you think the miniature poodle or the wire-haired terrier will make <u>their/its</u> owner proud by winning "Best in Show"?

9. <u>We/Us</u> and Rodney planned that practical joke for weeks.

10. No one really liked <u>their/his or her</u> picture in the yearbook.

11. All of the bands in the contest played <u>their/its</u> best songs.

12. Each of the dancers had <u>his or her/their</u> own special style.

13. After my brother and I painted our parents' house, they divided the pay evenly between <u>him/he</u> and <u>me/I</u>.

14. Representatives of Computer Systems Inc. will be on campus tomorrow so that <u>they/it</u> can recruit recent graduates for <u>their/its</u> training program.

15. In every math course we've taken, Sara has gotten a higher grade than <u>I/me</u>.

16. Not one of the boys would admit <u>his/their</u> fear as we prepared for our first bungee jump.

17. <u>We/Us</u> two guys have been friends since the third grade.

18. If one wish had been granted to my father and <u>I/me</u>, we would have spent the rest of our lives fishing.

19. Hiking up the mountain made Raoul and <u>I/me</u> very tired, but we were glad we did it.

20. It would have been better for both <u>he/him</u> and <u>she/her</u> if they had discussed their problem with a counselor.

◆ 19.2 Pronouns

The following passage contains errors in the use of pronouns. Edit it to eliminate errors in pronoun case, pronoun-antecedent agreement, and reflexive pronoun forms. Also eliminate nonspecific and unnecessary pronouns.

Everyone is aware of the importance of exercise in maintaining their health. School children exercise theirselves once they are let loose in the schoolyard at recess. Many older children become involved in organized sports, so that team workouts and games become his or her exercise program. And, of course, us adults fill gyms and fitness centers to keep our bodies strong and fit.

However, exercise for babies, toddlers, and preschoolers is often ignored. Parents assume they get enough exercise by theirselves. When a parent or caretaker is busy, they may keep a baby or toddler confined in their stroller, baby seat, or play pen for too long. But, every young child needs exercise, or they may not develop at a normal rate. They recommend that caregivers involve even very young children in fun physical activities in order to keep they healthy.

My wife and me have spent time exercising our daughter Erin since she was a baby. Because Erin spent time on a blanket on the floor instead of in a play pen or bouncy seat, the baby got a lot of practice rolling her over. Erin and I, we played endless games of "pattycake" and "peekaboo." When Erin was a toddler, they told us that toddlers should have at least 30 minutes of physical activity spread through-out the day. During these play periods, we got she to move along with a song or play ball with we. I threw soft balls that her caught and threw back. Now Erin is a 9-year-old who can pitch for their baseball team. Our doctor also recommended that Erin have "free play" time for she to explore, push, and pull objects as well as balancing and climbing on safe surfaces. All this hard work has given we a healthy, energetic child.

◆ 20.1 Adjectives and Adverbs

In the following sentences, circle the correct adjective or adverb form in each of the underlined pairs.

1. The <u>funniest/most funniest</u> joke of all was told by an 8-year-old boy.

2. Colleen wasn't feeling <u>well/good</u> when she took the test, which was why she didn't do <u>well/good</u>.

3. The <u>wisest/most wise</u> piece of advice I ever got was to be true to myself.

4. Ali was a <u>better/more better</u> runner than his brother Hakim.

5. Which of these three necklaces looks <u>best/better</u> with this dress?

6. His parents were <u>real/really</u> angry when he looked them <u>direct/directly</u> in the eyes and lied.

7. We all felt <u>bad/badly</u> when the movie star treated her fan <u>bad/badly</u>.

8. Are you <u>full, fully</u> aware of the dangers in the plan you propose?

9. Which would make you feel <u>worse/worser</u>: doing something you want to do but fear or not doing it?

10. In choosing between physics and biology, Ruby decided that biology would be the <u>easier/easiest</u> subject for her to get an A in.

11. <u>This/These</u> tie and <u>that/those</u> shirt were meant for each other.

12. Lourdes never wanted anything <u>more strong/more strongly</u> than she wanted the leading role in the play.

13. If we don't get out of this store <u>quick/quickly</u>, I'm going to spend more money than I should.

14. Our washing machine hasn't been working too <u>well/good</u> and needs to be replaced by one that works <u>better/more good</u>.

15. The <u>healthier/more healthier</u> plan is to include some fat in one's diet, while a no-fat diet is <u>dangerouser/more dangerous</u>.

16. On a blind date, <u>this/these</u> woman and <u>that/those</u> man may like each other, or they may not.

17. I thought nothing could be <u>worse/worst</u> than not having a date for New Year's Eve until I was fixed up with the <u>worse/worst</u> blind date of my life.

18. Barbara Kingsolver is a <u>well/good</u> novelist who writes <u>well/good</u> about current problems in society.

19. We considered each person's opinion because <u>this/these</u> or <u>that/those</u> idea might turn out to be the solution.

20. In our creative writing class, we try to treat each writer <u>good/well</u> whether or not we think the person's story or poem is a <u>good/well</u> one.

◆ 20.2 Adjectives and Adverbs

Edit the following passage to eliminate errors in the use of adjectives and adverbs.

(1) The sport of ice climbing has become real popular in recent years. (2) Most ice climbers try this sport after mastering rock climbing, which is the easiest of the two. (3) Climbing an icy slope is dangerouser than climbing a mountain in more warm weather. (4) In order to do good at ice climbing, you need to first gain experience climbing solider rocks.

(5) Enthusiasts say that they love the physical and mental challenge of climbing in freezing and often wet weather on more slipperier surfaces. (6) Many say the ice is more beautifuller than anything they have ever seen. (7) Some say they like being more scareder than they have ever been too. (8) Ice climbers progress from climbing mountain slopes of 45 degrees to challenginger frozen waterfalls that are almost vertical sheets of ice.

(9) However, the sport has become more safer in recent years. (10) This is the result of more better equipment and climbing techniques. (11) Climbers wear plastic or insulated leather boots with crampons attached to the bottom. (12) These crampons have 10 or 12 metal "teeth" that help feet grip the ice more tight. (13) In a technique called "top-roping," a metal connector is planted secure at the top of the climbing surface, and a rope is hung from it. (14) This feat is done by the experiencedest climber in the group. (15) Those climber makes his or her way up the ice by driving an axe or pick into the ice. (16) Climbers use their boots and crampons to gain footholds in the ice. (17) This actions are made safer because climbers wear harnesses that are attached to the rope held in place by the connector at the top. (18) The best ice climbers use deliberately moves to climb efficient up the ice. (19) Beginners are usually wastefuller of their energy. (20) They climb too forceful and get tired too quick.

◆ 21.1 Grammar and Usage Issues for ESL Writers

Rewrite each of the following sentences to add missing words, to delete unneeded pronouns and articles, to replace words used incorrectly, and to correct errrors in word order.

1. Wasn't a good idea.

    _____

2. She learned to play golf so could join her husband on weekends.

    _____

3. My brother he went back to Afghanistan to teach school.

    _____

4. When a rap song blasted on the radio, song woke Hiroshi from a deep sleep.

    _____

5. The worst experience I ever had, I was separated from my family for a year and didn't know where they were.

    _____

6. The children brought a lot of sands into the house from the beach outside.

    _____

7. I received ten mails today.

    _____

8. Margit drinks her tea with two sugars and a few milk.

    _____

9. Are many obstacles to finding a suitable place to live.

    _____

10. If there are the chocolate cookies around, I can't eat one cookie and stop there.

    _____

11. Most people need the routine as well as the stimulation in their lives.

    _____

12. Siri and her family live on the Montgomery Street near the East Side Highway.

    _____

13. Our school library has much computers available to students.

_____

14. Red-haired both twin boys have freckled faces.

_____

15. Please don't worry that problem about.

_____

16. Is teaching the class tomorrow who?

_____

17. The engine is needing some oil or it won't run well.

_____

18. That orange broken-down ugly reclining chair should be thrown out.

_____

19. The charity was grateful at our large donation.

_____

20. Our lawyer objected with the judge's decision.

_____

◆ 21.2 Grammar and Usage Issues for ESL Writers

Read the following essay, which contains errors in the use of subjects, verbs, determiners, articles, and prepositions in familiar expressions. All sentences have one or two errors. If a word or phrase is incorrect, cross it out and write the correction above the line. If a word is missing, add it on the line above.

(1) Last year, I moved from my noisy city neighborhood to small house on quiet country road. (2) I knew my new life would contrast from my old one. (3) Didn't realize how different would be. (4) At first, quiet of the country bothered me. (5) First night I was in my new home, I was hearing strange noises outside. (6) Were loud noises like singing all night. (7) The next day, I learned that these noises were made by much tiny frogs called "peepers."

(8) In my city apartment building, I didn't have many contact with my neighbors. (9) But, on my country road, my next-door neighbors made sure that I became acquainted to them. (10) They invited me for coffee and the pie. (11) I was grateful to their friendliness. (12) In fact, now are good friends. (13) We depend with each other for small favors, like watching each other's pets when we are away.

(14) Life in my small country town differs with city life in much ways. (15) I can take advantage with many outdoor activities. (16) Much months of the year, I am busy in my garden. (17) Are many places to swim, hike, climb mountains, and ride a bicycle. (18) I am also pleased from the spirit in my home town. (19) Everyone works together to protect the nature against the destruction. (20) When city friends ask me if I'm bored to living in a small country town, I reply, "No way!"

◆ 22.1 Using Commas

Add commas to the following sentences as necessary to set off items in series, introductory phrases, appositives, and transitional and parenthetical words, as well as in dates and place names. If any sentences are correct as written, write *C* in the blank.

1. Joan Kroc widow of the founder of McDonald's hamburger restaurants gives generously to many causes. _____

2. In fact she is one of the top philanthropists in America. _____

3. She has contributed over $150 million dollars to help the disadvantaged heal the sick house the homeless and promote world peace. _____

4. In 1982, the year her husband died Mrs. Kroc founded Ronald McDonald House Charities. _____

5. Named after the famous clown Ronald McDonald Houses are residences near hospitals where families of seriously ill children can stay. _____

6. Over the years Joan Kroc has donated more than $100 million dollars to this foundation. _____

7. Today the organization sponsors children's health charities in 32 countries. _____

8. Much of her giving however, is closer to home. _____

9. Mrs. Kroc is a resident of San Diego California. _____

10. After witnessing the poverty in southeast San Diego Joan Kroc donated 80 million dollars to the Salvation Army to build a community center there. _____

11. Currently the center provides local children with before- and after-school programs in academic subjects sports and creative and performing arts such as music acting art and dancing. _____

12. The center a large complex includes a gymnasium a 500-seat theater, a library filled with computers, a swimming pool, an ice skating rink and facilities for a variety of sports. _____

13. The center also provides child care, as well as family counseling and services for the elderly. _____

14. In addition Mrs. Kroc has donated money to help flood victims in Grand Forks North Dakota to AIDS research and to rehabilitation programs. _____

15. Recently Joan Kroc has focused her giving on the issue of world peace. _____

16. She donated 6 million dollars to the University of Notre Dame to establish an Institute for International Peace Studies where hopefully, workable plans for world peace can be created. _____

17. A few years later she founded the Kroc Institute for Peace and Justice at the University of San Diego. _____

18. At the Institute political leaders, scholars students and activists gather to work together in the cause of peace. _____

19. In response to the attacks of September 11 2001 both institutes are busier than ever. _____

20. Joan Kroc, a person who cares about peace is making a contribution toward a better future for everyone. _____

◆ 22.2 Using Commas

Add commas to the following paragraph as necessary to set off items in series, introductory phrases, appositives, and transitional and parenthetical words, as well as in dates and place names.

(1) To scientists a fossil is not just the remains of a long-dead plant or animal. (2) The name *trace fossil* can be given to any evidence that living creatures were once in a particular area. (3) For example dinosaur footprints are just as much fossils as dinosaur bones and teeth. (4) Worms burrowed through soil millions of years ago claim experts. (5) Tunnels in the soil now hardened into rock reveal what the worms were like. (6) Molds another type of trace fossil are formed when bones shells and other hard materials make an imprint in mud. (7) These molds show what the animal or plant looked like even without remains.

(8) Fossils are most often found in layers of rock that were formed from sand mud shells and other materials. (9) Over thousands of years water washes over buried objects like bones teeth and shells in the ground. (10) Minerals from the water gradually replace all or part of the object creating a hard fossil. (11) As time goes by that fossil becomes embedded in the rock.

(12) Paleontologists scientists who study ancient forms of life get a lot of information from fossils. (13) For instance they can figure out from an animal's footprint how tall it was how much it weighed and how it moved around. (14) Animal droppings can tell what the creature ate. (15) The most revealing fossils are bodies of animals that have dried out in the desert or were preserved in ice or tar. (16) For this reason we know what woolly mammoths shaggy elephant-like beasts from over a million years ago looked like. (17) The La Brea tar pits in Los Angeles California became a burial place for many Ice Age animals. (18) The bones of saber-toothed tigers giant ground sloths and mammoths have all been found in the tar pits. (19) The George C. Page Museum right near the tar pits contains skeletons of these animals. (20) Since 1906 scientists have been studying these remains.

◆ 23.1 Using Apostrophes

Edit the following sentences to eliminate errors in the use of apostrophes. Look for apostrophes that need to be added, deleted, or put in another place in the word. If any sentences are correct as written, write *C* in the blank.

1. The New York City firefighters bravery brought them national recognition.

   _____

2. You wo'nt believe the story I just heard. _____

3. Everyone says thats not what happened. _____

4. Their apartment is identical in size and layout to our's. _____

5. Lois's clothes are always appropriate for the occasion. _____

6. Womens' fashions can change drastically from year to year, while mens'

   remain pretty much the same. _____

7. Whos in charge of payroll at this company? _____

8. The girls' carefully stored their hockey equipment after the game. _____

9. I'm afraid we'll have to charge you for that broken vase. _____

10. The Riveras house is right next door to their's. _____

11. The school board gave all the principal's a raise. _____

12. Lets find out if this lost handbag is her's. _____

13. The entire class's test scores have gone up since the beginning of the semester.

    _____

14. Wouldnt it be better to buy those sneakers on sale? _____

15. John Adams's son, John Quincy Adams, was this countrys' sixth president.

    _____

16. A knights' suit of armor protected the warrior's entire body. _____

17. Sandra Cisneros' stories of Hispanic life always touch my heart. _____

18. Its fun to watch the kitten play with it's toy. _____

19. If everybody tried to understand the beliefs of other's, we'd all get along better.

    _____

20. The business' profits have gone up but its stock has not done the same. _____

◆ 23.2 Using Apostrophes

Edit the following passage to eliminate errors in the use of apostrophes. Look for apostrophes that need to be added, deleted, or put in a different place in the word.

(1) Many peoples' reaction to a dentists' chair is one of fear. (2) One dentist estimates that over 90 percent of her patients are afraid of dental work. (3) "Sometimes they'll get nervous just hearing the drill," she says, "even when the teeth being drilled are'nt their's. (4). . . I've been bitten a lot, too, and most of the time its an accident," she asserts. (5) But she also suspects that a few bites have been on purpose. (6) Because this dentist is a wholesome-looking young woman, patients have told her, "You dont look like someone whod be a dentist." (7) Its even worse when they find out that she's a specialist in root canals.

(8) Our teeths' tendency to decay has caused painful problems for millions of years. (9) In prehistoric times, there was'nt much to do but pull out a rotted tooth. (10) Later, wealthy Egyptians, Greeks, and Romans of ancient times' could replace their teeth with fake gold ones. (11) The jewelers' skill was employed to make false teeth in the Middle Ages. (12) However, pulling teeth was usually the barber's job. (13) Later, surgeons' took over. (14) A French dental scientist, Pierre Fauchard, published a treatise called *The Surgeon Dentist* in 1728. (15) The book's illustrations showed dental tools and devices of the time. (16) In 1840, the worlds' first dental school opened its doors in Baltimore, Maryland. (17) Heres what a visit to the dentist's office would have been like around 1850. (18) Ether or nitrous oxide wouldve been used to make you unconscious before painful procedures. (19) Now there are local anesthetics' that block pain only in the area the dentist is working on. (20) Let's all be thankful for the advances that minimize pain in modern dentistry.

◆ 24.1 Understanding Mechanics

Edit the following sentences to eliminate errors in capitalization of common and proper nouns, punctuation of direct quotations, and title format. If any sentences are correct as written, write *C* in the blank.

1. "I am still skeptical about this new discovery, said the scientist from princeton university. _____

2. Joelle's Math class meets tuesday afternoon in olin hall. _____

3. Jerry Seinfeld was a popular Comedian even before he starred in the television series *seinfeld*. _____

4. Many muslims make a pilgrimage to Mecca in saudi arabia as part of their religious practice. _____

5. The writer annie dillard said, The secret of seeing is to sail on solar wind.

   _____

6. Some of the chinese-american characters in Amy Tan's book "The Joy Luck Club" live on Sacramento street. _____

7. My brother Louis, who joined the boy scouts in February, said that "he looks forward to hiking and camping at the lake near our town." _____

8. In his poem The Waste Land, t. s. Eliot wrote, April is the cruelest month.

   _____

9. A story in "Time" magazine praised Denzel Washington's performance as a civil rights Leader in the movie malcolm x. _____

10. The computer company Microsoft, which developed the program microsoft explorer, is located East of seattle in redmond, washington. _____

11. In history 111, we studied the revolutionary war and the United States constitution. _____

12. The jewish holiday of Passover, which takes place in the Spring, includes many special foods. _____

13. You may know that uncle Robert, who can speak both english and french, is fond of saying, "speaking two languages is like having two minds". _____

14. The department of environmental conservation is responsible for protecting natural resources such as Rivers and Forests. _____

15. In The Wizard of Oz, dorothy clicks her heels together and says, there's no place like home. _____

16. Like many who held the office before him, president George w. Bush was once a state Governor. _____

17. The centerville garden club meets the first Tuesday of every month except in Winter. _____

18. "If we are going to be the next ford motor company, said the Manager, employees will have to be here on time Monday morning." _____

19. The americans and the japanese fought some of the second world war's fiercest battles on Islands in the pacific ocean. _____

20. The women's softball team plays Marilyn Monroe's song "Diamonds Are a Girl's Best Friend" at every game. _____

◆ 24.2 Understanding Mechanics

Edit the following passage to eliminate errors in capitalization of common and proper nouns, punctuation of direct quotations, and title format.

(1) There is a long tradition of travel in the united states. (2) For one thing, the Nation is made up of people from other places, including europe, africa, and asia. (3) The earliest Settlers landed on the shores of what are now massachusetts and virginia. (4) It did not take long for the mostly english settlers to found cities such as boston and philadelphia. (5) They also built Harvard university, which was originally a christian college.

(6) Throughout their history, americans have been restless. (7) "Go west, young man, is a famous quotation from the Nation's pioneer days. (8) People crossed the mississippi river in great numbers to establish farms and Businesses. (9) They encountered driving snow in january and february and intense heat in Summer. (10) Still, many succeeded in reaching the west.

(11) Today, people travel to see the country and its best known places, including the statue of liberty in New York city and Bourbon street in new Orleans. (12) The American association for retired persons and similar Groups organize trips and tours. (13) The "new york times" and other newspapers have travel sections, with articles such as *Finding the best hotel in Minneapolis*. (14) The week after Christmas is an especially popular time to travel, when people visit uncle Bob and aunt Sue or go skiing in the rocky mountains. (15) "The winter is the best time to travel, one Travel Agent said, because most people need a change at that time of year".

(16) Many stories have been written about travel, including Jack Kerouac's book On the road. (17) Woody guthrie wrote a famous song about places in the united states. (18) In it, he sang, this land was made for you and me. (19) That

statement is still true today, as people travel from the Pacific ocean to the Atlantic ocean, perhaps hearing spanish spoken in houston and chinese in chicago. (20) No class in History or Geography could be as rewarding as seeing america's Deserts, rivers, mountains, and people firsthand.

◆ 25.1 Understanding Spelling

Edit the following sentences to eliminate spelling errors. Decide whether each underlined word is spelled correctly or incorrectly. If the word is misspelled, correct it in the space above. If the spelling given is correct, write *C* above the word.

1. The couch was the only <u>peice</u> of furniture my <u>roomate</u> and I bought together.

2. Six months after it opened, the <u>resterant</u> is finally <u>begining</u> to make money.

3. Although not <u>evryone</u> is afraid of <u>heights</u>, most people are <u>carefull</u> when they climb a ladder.

4. A fan sometimes <u>overates</u> the <u>actting</u> ability of her favorite movie star.

5. The failure of our elected leaders to <u>cooperate</u> with one another is <u>sensless</u>.

6. After the verdict was announced, the defendant's <u>releif</u> was <u>noticeable</u>.

7. Despite her <u>intelligence</u>, Joy is usually <u>embarassed</u> when she <u>trys</u> something new.

8. The <u>driness</u> of the soil made <u>diging</u> in the garden difficult.

9. Raphael <u>paid</u> <u>alot</u> more for his car <u>insureance</u> than he spent on the car itself.

10. The agent who <u>spyed</u> for the enemy did a <u>disservice</u> to his own <u>goverment</u>.

11. No one was <u>suprised</u> when Jaden, who could <u>describe</u> things well, <u>exceled</u> at <u>writeing</u> short stories.

12. As part of the restoration, the <u>cieling</u> of the theater near the <u>entrence</u> was <u>finally</u> repainted.

13. Many men and <u>woman</u> left Ireland and came to the United States when a blight <u>destroyed</u> much of Ireland's <u>potatoe</u> crop.

14. The <u>neighbors'</u> new dog is young and <u>plaiful</u>.

15. The <u>arguement</u> lasted from <u>Wensday</u> to Sunday.

16. After she had <u>climbed</u> to the top of the mountain, Michelle was <u>disatisfied</u> with the view.

17. My <u>freind</u> Sam is <u>probly</u> one of the best <u>runers</u> in the school.

18. Understanding <u>grammer</u> can make <u>createing</u> a <u>sentence</u> much more <u>intresting</u>.

19. Nothing <u>occured</u> in the office that the <u>secretary</u> did not know about.

20. There is <u>generaly</u> a great deal of <u>excitement</u> when an important question is <u>answerred</u> by <u>sceintists</u>.

◆ 25.2 Understanding Spelling

Edit the following sentences to eliminate spelling errors. Correct each misspelled word in the space above it.

(1) Do you know for certian what time it is? (2) Luckily, modern cultures have developed definate ways of keeping track of time. (3) But can you imagine never nowing the time of day, or even the month of the year?

(4) That describes the life of many erly peoples. (5) Though anceint cultures were dependant on farming for their livelyhood, farmers sometimes had trouble deciding when to plant and harvest. (6) That was because few noticable signs occured to tell farmers that planting time had arrived. (7) The Mayans were among the first to make a truely advanced calender for measuring the seasons. (8) They based it in part on the placment of the stars at different times of the year.

(9) Another tool used before the begining of modern times was the sundial. (10) The sundial displaied the time of day in the form of a shadow. (11) As the sun climed in the sky, the shadow moved across the sundial to show the hour. (12) Yet it was not possible to know the time to the minuet, and a sundial only worked untill the sun went down at night. (13) Therefore, people had to use a great deal of judgement in planing their daily activities.

(14) The first clocks made it easier to measure tinyer amounts of time. (15) Finaly, everyone knew when it was exactly fourty minutes past eight o'clock. (16) Soon, more events began happenning during the day, and life started becoming busier.

(17) While clocks were an improvement, they destroied a slower, more liesurely way of life. (18) Because time has become so easy to measure, most people now beleive that events should begin at specific times, and they consider any lateness to be an annoyance. (19) Such people would argue that strict time keeping has simpley made things better. (20) Yet others feel that our crowded schedules have taken some of the enjoiment out of life.

◆ 26.1 Learning Commonly Confused Words

Edit the following sentences to eliminate errors in the use of commonly confused words. Decide whether each underlined word is used correctly or incorrectly. If the word is used incorrectly, correct it in the space above. If the word is used correctly, write *C* above the word.

1. When the actor <u>excepted</u> the award, he said that it was <u>quit</u> an honor.

2. Researchers believe that babies benefit when they <u>here</u> <u>fine</u> music before <u>their</u> born.

3. A <u>lose</u> muffler can have a serious <u>affect</u> on the amount of noise a car makes.

4. I always ignore the fancier <u>desserts</u> and order a piece of <u>plane</u> apple pie because <u>its</u> my favorite.

5. The <u>principle</u> of the school asked the students to <u>set</u> <u>quitely</u> during the assembly.

6. As long as Rodrigo keeps his keys on the table <u>buy</u> the door, he will always <u>know</u> <u>wear</u> they are.

7. Employees are not <u>suppose</u> to make personal calls during work hours <u>accept</u> when there is an emergency.

8. Even when a person is not <u>conscience</u> and alert, the person's <u>mine</u> is active, taking in information and controlling the body's functions.

9. Philip <u>set</u> his coffee mug on the roof of his car and <u>than</u> remembered it just as he released the parking <u>break</u>.

10. The shortstop <u>through</u> the ball to first <u>base</u> more <u>then</u> 50 times during practice.

11. On the first day of class, the instructor said, "I trust that everyone <u>hear</u> has <u>all</u> <u>ready</u> purchased the textbook for the <u>course</u>."

12. Our cottage at the lake is so <u>peaceful</u> that I can <u>lay</u> in the hammock for hours with <u>know</u> interruptions.

13. Teddy cannot use an expensive gadget without <u>braking</u> it.

14. The experienced shopper <u>new</u> it was more economical to <u>by</u> a gallon of milk than it was to get <u>too</u> smaller cartons.

15. The young women were <u>already</u> to <u>quit</u> their jobs in order to become famous musicians.

16. The officer could <u>fine</u> no reason to <u>suppose</u> that the suspect's statement was false.

17. Frederick <u>past</u> the exam by cheating, but his <u>conscious</u> bothered him so much that he confessed to the dean.

18. That cat <u>lays</u> around <u>everyday</u> and does nothing.

19. If you plan to wash <u>you're</u> car today, <u>would</u> you please wash mine, <u>to</u>?

20. In the <u>passed</u>, people <u>use</u> to <u>write</u> letters more often.

◆ 26.2 Learning Commonly Confused Words

Edit the following sentences to eliminate errors in the use of commonly confused words. Correct each improperly used word in the space above it.

(1) Carnival season is a time too celebrate in many cities around the world. (2) During carnival, people sit aside their every day routines. (3) Instead, they fine ways to enjoy themselves before the quite season of Lent.

(4) At carnival time, many people by costumes to wear at parades and per-formances. (5) Traditionally, each person is suppose to choose a costume that is the opposite of what he or she is use to wearing. (6) For example, someone whose ordinarily dressed in plane clothes might wear a costume that is bright and showy. (7) Women create dramatic affects with feathers and high headdresses, while men wear masks or face paint so know one will recognize them.

(8) The strangely dressed people than fill the streets to here wonderful music. (9) One of the principle activities of carnival is dancing. (10) Men and women recreate dances from the passed that rise the spirits of all who see them. (11) Also important during carnival are the find parades that are staged by competing groups. (12) People set on beautifully decorated floats and throw beads and lose candy to spectators. (13) Later, children often complain that people on the floats through all the candy to the wrong part of the crowd—the section were they stood being the write part, of course.

(14) Carnival ends in Mardi Gras, or Fat Tuesday, when groups give they're most impressive parades and performances. (15) Then comes Lent, a season of pieceful fasting and prayer. (16) After all that celebration, its time to prepare for the Easter holiday.

Answers

Sentence Skills Diagnostic Test

	Answer	Skill or problem	*Foundations First* chapter	Exercise Central exercises
1.	a	sentence fragments	12	629, 630, 631, 632
2.	a	subject-verb agreement	13	633, 634, 635, 636, 637, 638, 639
3.	a	illogical shifts	14	640, 641, 642
4.	a	dangling and misplaced modifiers	15	643, 644, 645, 646
5.	b	verbs: past tense	16	647, 648, 649, 650
6.	c	nouns and pronouns	18–19	658, 659, 660, 661, 662, 663, 664, 665, 666, 667, 668
7.	a	adjectives and adverbs	20	669, 670, 671, 672, 673
8.	a	ESL issues	21	674, 675, 676, 677, 678, 679, 680, 681
9.	a	commas	22	682, 683, 684, 685, 686, 687, 688
10.	a	apostrophes	23	689, 690, 691
11.	b	parallelism	10	625, 626
12.	a	run-ons and comma splices	11	627, 628
13.	b	ESL issues	21	674, 675, 676, 677, 678, 679, 680, 681
14.	c	illogical shifts	14	640, 641, 642
15.	a	subject-verb agreement	13	633, 634, 635, 636, 637, 638, 639
16.	c	commas	22	682, 683, 684, 685, 686, 687, 688
17.	b	mechanics	24	692, 693, 694
18.	b	parallelism	10	625, 626
19.	b	ESL issues	21	674, 675, 676, 677, 678, 679, 680, 681
20.	a	apostrophes	23	689, 690, 691
21.	b	run-ons and comma splices	11	627, 628

	Answer	Skill or problem	*Foundations First* chapter	Exercise Central exercises
22.	b	sentence fragments	12	629, 630, 631, 632
23.	a	illogical shifts	14	640, 641, 642
24.	c	verbs: past tense	16	647, 648, 649, 650
25.	a	nouns and pronouns	18–19	658, 659, 660, 661, 662, 663, 664, 665, 666, 667, 668
26.	a	adjectives and adverbs	20	669, 670, 671, 672, 673
27.	b	verbs: past participles	17	651, 652, 653, 654, 655, 656, 657
28.	c	ESL issues	21	674, 675, 676, 677, 678, 679, 680, 681
29.	c	parallelism	10	625, 626
30.	c	subject-verb agreement	13	633, 634, 635, 636, 637, 638, 639
31.	c	commas	22	682, 683, 684, 685, 686, 687, 688
32.	b	mechanics	24	692, 693, 694
33.	c	run-ons and comma splices	11	627, 628
34.	c	illogical shifts	14	640, 641, 642
35.	b	sentence fragments	12	629, 630, 631, 632
36.	a	verbs: past tense	16	647, 648, 649, 650
37.	b	nouns and pronouns	18–19	658, 659, 660, 661, 662, 663, 664, 665, 666, 667, 668
38.	a	ESL issues	21	674, 675, 676, 677, 678, 679, 680, 681
39.	a	commas	22	682, 683, 684, 685, 686, 687, 688
40.	a	subject-verb agreement	13	633, 634, 635, 636, 637, 638, 639
41.	b	dangling and misplaced modifiers	15	643, 644, 645, 646
42.	c	verbs: past participles	17	651, 652, 653, 654, 655, 656, 657
43.	b	ESL issues	21	674, 675, 676, 677, 678, 679, 680, 681
44.	c	nouns and pronouns	18–19	658, 659, 660, 661, 662, 663, 664, 665, 666, 667, 668
45.	c	ESL issues	21	674, 675, 676, 677, 678, 679, 680, 681
46.	b	adjectives and adverbs	20	669, 670, 671, 672, 673
47.	c	illogical shifts	14	640, 641, 642

Answer	Skill or problem	*Foundations First* chapter	Exercise Central exercises
48. b	subject-verb agreement	13	633, 634, 635, 636, 637, 638, 639
49. a	dangling and misplaced modifiers	15	643, 644, 645, 646
50. c	ESL issues	21	674, 675, 676, 677, 678, 679, 680, 681

◆ 6.1 Writing Simple Sentences

Answers: **1.** Complete subject: A caterpillar; complete verb: spun; prepositional phrases: on a milkweed stalk, beside the road; simple subject: caterpillar; action verb: spun. **2.** Complete subject: Our bathroom window; complete verb: is allowing; prepositional phrases: into the wall, above the bathtub; simple subject: window; action verb: allowing. **3.** Complete subject: Howard; complete verb: doesn't know; prepositional phrases: After reading six novels, about the British navy, from a schooner; simple subject: Howard; action verb: know. **4.** Complete subject: tornado; complete verb: flattened; prepositional phrases: On the other side, of the valley; simple subject: tornado; action verb: flattened. **5.** Complete subject: The F.B.I. agents standing in the doorway; complete verb: were making; prepositional phrase: in the doorway; simple subject: agents; action verb: making. **6.** Complete subject: you; complete verb: can understand; prepositional phrases: to the opinions, on this Web site; simple subject: you; action verb: understand. **7.** Complete subject: The runt of the litter; complete verb: looked; prepositional phrase: of the litter; simple subject: runt; linking verb: looked. **8.** Complete subject: The campsites on the map of this national forest; complete verb; seem; prepositional phrases: on the map, of this national forest, from the highway; simple subject: campsites; linking verb: seem. **9.** Complete subject: everyone in the dorm; complete verb: has considered; prepositional phrase: Since his birthday party, in the dorm; simple subject: everyone; simple verb: considered. **10.** Complete subject: The smallest variety of lizard; complete verb: is; prepositional phrases: about the size, of a dime; simple subject: variety; linking verb: is. **11.** Complete subject: the shouting protesters outside City Hall; complete verb: collapsed; prepositional phrases: with arrest, outside City Hall, onto the sidewalk; simple subject: protesters; action verb: collapsed. **12.** Complete subject: The new administration's candidates for cabinet posts; complete verb: have been; prepositional phrases: for cabinet posts, without government experience; simple subject: candidates; linking verb: been. **13.** Complete subject: The horses at the hitching post outside the saloon; complete verb: waited; prepositional phrases: at the hitching post, outside the saloon, for their riders' return; simple subject: horses; action verb: waited. **14.** Complete subject: environmental issues and the economy; complete verb: appear; prepositional phrases: In an election year, to many politicians; simple subjects: issues, economy; linking verb: appear. **15.** Complete subject: The odd-looking bald man and his clever dog; complete verb: are; simple subjects: man, dog; linking verb: are. **16.** Complete subject: The sun lamp; complete verb: turned; prepositional phrase: of the patrons; simple subject: lamp; action verb: turned. **17.** Complete subject: Kathy; complete verb: wore; prepositional phrase: for the big day; simple subject: Kathy; action verb: wore. **18.** Complete subject: my strong-willed aunt; complete verb: was; prepositional phrases: After the stroke, in her recovery; simple subject: aunt; linking verb: was. **19.** Complete subject: A patent or other government license; complete verb: does guarantee; prepositional phrase: of vitamins and herbal supplements; simple subjects: patent, license; action verb: guarantee. **20.** Complete subject: hundreds of tourists outside the mouth of the cave; complete verb: watched; prepositional phrases: At dusk, of tourists, outside the mouth, of the cave, of the bats; simple subject: hundreds; action verb: watched.

◆ **6.2** **Writing Simple Sentences**

Answers: **1.** Complete subject: The peanut butter in the cupboard; complete verb: has become; prepositional phrase: in the cupboard; simple subject: butter; linking verb: become. **2.** Complete subject: One of the children; complete verb: has thrown; prepositional phrases: of the children, into the wastebasket; simple subject: One; action verb: thrown. **3.** Complete subject: the youngest girl; complete verb: announced; prepositional phrases: After lunch, for cheese sandwiches; simple subject: girl; action verb: announced. **4.** Complete subject: all three teachers at the preschool; complete verb; would agree; prepositional phrases: at the preschool, with her; simple subject: teachers; action verb: agree. **5.** Complete subject: napping; complete verb: does come; prepositional phrases: To the children, at the preschool; simple subject: napping; action verb: come. **6.** Complete subject: They; complete verb: are; prepositional phrase: about the other children and the toys; simple subject: They; linking verb: are. **7.** Complete subject: the adults; complete verb: have counted; prepositional phrases: on nap time, for cleaning up; simple subject: adults; action verb: counted. **8.** Complete subject: Jelly-covered fingers; complete verb: leave; prepositional phrase: on the walls and furniture; simple subject: fingers; action verb: leave. **9.** Complete subject: Emily; complete verb: has been spending; prepositional phrases: in day care, since a month, after her birth; simple subject: Emily; action verb: spending. **10.** Complete subject: Her younger brother and sister; complete verb: will be attending; simple subjects: brother, sister; action verb: attending. **11.** Complete subject: Everyone at preschool, including the teachers; complete verb: sings; prepositional phrases: at preschool, including the teachers, with gusto, during music time; simple subject: Everyone; action verb: sings. **12.** Complete subject: A college degree and current information about early childhood development; complete verb: are; prepositional phrases: about early childhood development, for this type, of work; simple subjects: degree, information; linking verb: are. **13.** Complete subject: the rewards of playing and singing with little boys and girls; complete verb: are; prepositional phrases: of playing and singing, with little boys and girls, for most people; simple subject: rewards; linking verb: are. **14.** Complete subject: A job working with infants and toddlers; complete verb: seems; prepositional phrases: with infants and toddlers, for some adults; simple subject: job; linking verb: seems. **15.** Complete subject: childcare providers; complete verb: receive; prepositional phrase: In the United States; simple subject: providers; action verb: receive. **16.** Complete subject: some extremely dedicated people; complete verb: go; prepositional phrases: With so few incentives, into the field, of child care; simple subject: people; action verb: go. **17.** Complete subject: some completely unqualified and uninterested people; complete verb: care; prepositional phrase: for young children; simple subject: people; action verb: care. **18.** Complete subject: Other countries; complete verb: make; prepositional phrases: by paying good wages, for the service; simple subject: Other countries; action verb: make. **19.** Complete subject: the welfare of children; complete verb: Should be; prepositional phrases: of children, to Americans, without young children, of their own; simple subject: welfare; linking verb: be. **20.** Complete subject: A good start in life; complete verb: can make; prepositional phrases: for the child, for the parents, for the rest, of society; simple subject: start; action verb: make.

◆ **7.1** **Writing Compound Sentences**

Suggested answers: (Other correct answers are possible.) **1.** The chicken flapped its wings, but it could not fly. **2.** The stapler did not work properly, so he opened it. **3.** My baby daughter cries frequently, for she cannot communicate with us any other way. **4.** He could not understand Arabic, nor could he read the French subtitles. **5.** You could change the opening paragraph, or you could just clarify the thesis statement. **6.** He went to clean the house on Friday, but the owners had forgotten to leave him a key. **7.** Pakistan has atomic weapons, and that fact frightens some people in India. **8.** Training a dog requires consistency, so the whole family should treat the dog the same way. **9.** The teacher was prepared for the lesson, and the students had done their homework. **10.** Punk rock continues to attract new fans, but it has been around for thirty years. **11.** Most cable television shows attract small audiences; however, many of the shows are well acted and well written. **12.** Carla's suitcase was not on her connecting flight; therefore, she arrived with only a toothbrush. **13.** The enchiladas were delicious; in fact, they tasted even better than my mother's. **14.** Marcus's company went out of business in May; nevertheless, he has managed to pay his rent on time. **15.** This letter to the editor contains some inaccurate information; for example, very few local people supported the council members' proposal. **16.** Tomas received the highest score on the midterm exam; in addition, he was on time for every class session. **17.** The public ignored the scandal; however, newspapers and television shows discussed nothing else. **18.** My credit card bills were breaking my budget; therefore, I had to stop using the cards. **19.** Every bite caused terrible pain in my tooth; still, I avoided seeing my dentist. **20.** Each year in the Chinese calendar is named for an animal; for example, this is the Year of the Ox.

◆ 7.2   Writing Compound Sentences

Suggested answers: (Other correct answers are possible)

a. **1.** Weather forecasters often get to appear on television, **2.** *and t*he job offers some prestige. **3.** Forecasting the weather seems like an attractive position to many Americans; **4.** *however,* weather forecasting does not seem so appealing in some other countries. **5.** A weatherman in Rio de Janeiro forecast rain on New Year's Eve. **6.** Continual rainstorms had dampened many Brazilians' spirits, **7.** *so m*any people simply stayed away from the outdoor celebration. **8.** The New Year's Eve party was a flop. **9.** The predicted rain never arrived; **10.** *subsequently, t*he weatherman was sent to jail for his mistake.

b. **1.** Asthma affects nine million American children. **2.** Smog has long been blamed for making the chronic illness worse; **3.** *however, p*oor air quality seems actually to cause asthma. **4.** A study followed children in twelve communities in southern California for ten years, **5.** *and t*he results were published in a respected medical journal. **6.** The children were reasonably healthy to begin with; **7.** *for example, a*ll participated in athletics. **8.** Six of the communities had fairly clean air, **9.** *but t*he rest had some of the poorest air quality in the United States. **10.** The children in smoggy areas were three to four times more likely to develop asthma.

◆ 8.1   Writing Complex Sentences

Suggested answers: (Other correct answers are possible.) **1.** Although I felt good about my performance on the test, I received only an average grade. **2.** Rajiv stopped delivery of his newspapers and mail before he went out of town for the weekend. **3.** While the employees were picketing outside the factory, the manager was training replacement workers. **4.** The fans stood and roared when the pitcher walked a third batter. **5.** She cleaned houses and offices until she finished her degree and went to law school. **6.** Because Andreas has a learning disability, he receives extra time for his examinations. **7.** After Beatrice spent the night watching over her sick son, she was exhausted. **8.** As one small boy watched, the other children played in the schoolyard. **9.** I took my car for a tuneup so that it will get me safely to my parents' house in Oklahoma. **10.** Since Huey has been living in the suburbs, he has found new pastimes. **11.** Ida Lupino, who acted in many well-known films, also earned respect as a director. **12.** My doctor, whose husband is an accountant, keeps her billing information in an old shoebox. **13.** The tree that hangs over his driveway stands on his neighbor's property. **14.** This old farm, which has been in Raul's family for decades, seldom makes a profit. **15.** Children who eat a lot of candy often get cavities. **16.** Internet stock prices, which had been unrealistically high, fell quickly. **17.** William Wegman, whose photographs of dogs made him famous, began taking pictures of his Weimaraner named Man Ray. **18.** The letter that is on the table has no return address. **19.** This office, which has no window, is the only available one on this floor. **20.** The centennial celebration for the town, which has a declining population, took place last year.

◆ 8.2   Writing Complex Sentences

Suggested answers: (Other correct answers are possible.) **1.** Harold Russell was working in a market in Massachusetts **2.** *when t*he United States entered World War II. **3.** Russell, *who* considered himself a failure, **4.** immediately enlisted in the army. **5.** Russell trained as a paratrooper. **6.** He also learned demolition, **7.** *which* earned him a position as an instructor. **8.** *As t*he D-Day invasion was taking place, **9.** Harold Russell was teaching soldiers in North Carolina. **10.** He was holding some TNT **11.** *that* turned out to have a faulty fuse. **12.** The bomb exploded in his hands, **13.** *which* had to be amputated and replaced with steel hooks.

14. *Because* Russell became extremely skilled at using the hooks, **15.** *he* made a training film for other disabled soldiers. **16.** The Hollywood director William Wyler, *who* saw the film, **17.** cast Russell in the movie *The Best Years of Our Lives*. **18.** *Although* Harold Russell had never acted in his life, **19.** *he* won the Oscar for best supporting actor in 1946. **20.** Russell then retired from acting to work for veterans' causes.

◆ 9.1   Fine-Tuning Your Sentences

Suggested answers: (Other correct answers are possible.) **1.** In the 1950s, smallpox was still infecting fifty million people a year. **2.** The World Health Organization campaigned to vaccinate as many people as possible. **3.** This deadly and disfiguring disease had disappeared by the 1970s. **4.** People around the world were supposedly safe from smallpox. **5.** As a result, vaccination against smallpox stopped.

6. The smallpox virus was stored in two places, top-security laboratories in Russia and one in the United States. **7.** Supposedly, no one but scientists had access to the virus. **8.** They studied the virus and ways to defeat it under secure and sterile conditions. **9.** The World Health Organization planned to destroy the remaining virus stocks in 1999 but changed the deadline to 2002. **10.** The virus was to be destroyed because then smallpox would no longer exist.

11. Health officials now suspect that terrorists could have the smallpox virus. **12.** Since 1979, no one in the United States has been vaccinated, and this poses a threat. **13.** The vaccination loses effectiveness after seven to ten years. **14.** Threats of bioterrorism have made people feel threatened and anxious. **15.** Unfortunately, the existing supply of the vaccine is small. **16.** Recent efforts to produce more vaccine have not yielded large amounts. **17.** A new, more powerful kind of smallpox vaccine is now being developed and tested. **18.** However, this process could take two or more years.

19. In 2002, the executive board of the World Health Organization recommended delaying the destruction of the virus because the virus can help to develop vaccines and cures. **20.** The organization wants research to proceed quickly. **21.** In 2004 or 2005, the members will review the smallpox situation again.

◆ 9.2   Fine-Tuning Your Sentences

Suggested answers: (Other correct answers are possible.) **1.** The ability to laugh makes us human. **2.** For centuries, people have believed this idea. **3.** Laughter may occur in animals other than human beings, however. **4.** According to some studies, dogs and even rats may be able to laugh.

5. A researcher named Patricia Simonet recorded the sounds of playing dogs. **6.** The dogs appeared to be panting normally. **7.** Later, Simonet and her students at Sierra Nevada College analyzed the recordings. **8.** They discovered that the pants covered more sound frequencies than normal panting does. **9.** Dogs in aggressive clashes did not pant in the same way. **10.** The research team wondered if the unusual panting could indicate that the dogs were laughing. **11.** When the team broadcast recordings of the dog "laughter" for other dogs, the dogs picked up toys and approached the sound, ready to play.

12. Rats may laugh, too. **13.** When they wrestle playfully with other rats, they chirp. **14.** They also chirp before mating or receiving morphine in laboratory tests. **15.** Brian Knutson of the National Institutes of Health recorded these sounds, and a second researcher, Jaak Panksepp of Bowling Green University, has recorded similar rat noises. **16.** Panksepp tickles the rats to make them chirp. **17.** He warns others, "You have to know the rat."

18. This research might sound silly except that testing animal laughter has a serious purpose. **19.** Through such research, neuroscientists can trace the way brains process rewards. **20.** Laughing dogs and rats may someday increase our understanding of how animals, including humans, communicate.

◆ 10.1   Using Parallelism

Suggested answers: (Other correct answers are possible.) **1.** You can either write a personal check or use cash at this restaurant. **2.** The band played too loudly and slowly. **3.** Some of the veterans walked briskly, some limped along, and some rode on a float. **4.** Being in good physical condition is more important for overall health than being thin. **5.** The food was greasy, salty, and delicious. **6.** His argument uses faulty logic, misleading statistics, and irrelevant examples. **7.** Correct **8.** *Beowulf* is written in Old English, *The Canterbury Tales* in Middle English, and Shakespeare's plays in an early form of modern English. **9.** Grandmother banded her hens with yellow rings and her pullets with red rings. **10.** The bathroom looked shabby because of the cracked tile, the rust-stained floor, and the mildewed grout. **11.** Phobias can make people afraid of open spaces or elevators. **12.** I wanted neither to go back home nor to stay there. **13.** Correct **14.** February has to be short because it is dreary, cold, and too close to spring. **15.** The speech was not only well written but also beautifully delivered. **16.** The sweet sixteen party of her dreams would feature a boy band, real flowers in crystal vases, and ballroom dancing. **17.** The pictures that accompany the recipes are out of focus, garishly tinted, and unappetizing. **18.** The dog trainer commanded the collie to heel, sit, and stay. **19.** The tune I heard might have come from a Broadway show or from a Beatles song. **20.** Correct

◆ 10.2   Using Parallelism

Suggested answers: (Other correct answers are possible.) **1.** For decades, people with low self-esteem were said to be likely to commit crimes, abuse drugs, and go to jail. **2.** Psychologists frequently blamed a decision to plant a bomb or beat a spouse on a lack of self-respect. **3.** Based on the results of psychological tests, schoolchildren were identified as either having confidence or lacking self-esteem. **4.** Experts wanted to protect children with low self-confidence from lives of misery and crime. **5.** Therefore, for the past twenty years, social workers, psychologists, and teachers have all been expected to help children develop a sense of self-worth.

6. But is low self-esteem really such a terrible problem? **7.** Everyone has met at least one person who both possesses plenty of self-confidence and treats other people badly. **8.** Since the first self-esteem tests were administered, young people have become ever more likely to get high scores than to perform poorly. **9.** However, crime rates, illegal drug use, and cruel treatment of other people have not improved in that time. **10.** Today, while many young people have high self-esteem, they may neither have good social skills nor do well in school.

11. Some psychologists have begun to think that high self-esteem either is not a huge influence on a person's quality of life or is actually a problem for some people. **12.** One researcher believes that people with low self-esteem not only may not be harmed by it, but may actually do better in school than more confident students. **13.** He says that students with low self-esteem study more and push themselves harder because they fear that they will not succeed. **14.** Another psychologist has found that people with high self-esteem are likely to hurt other people or endanger them. **15.** Furthermore, according to psychological research, people who are violent or racist do not secretly feel bad about themselves. **16.** One psychologist suggested that such people would be better off feeling worse about themselves than feeling better.

17. At any rate, many psychologists now believe that feeling bad about oneself does not cause terrorism, substance abuse, and reckless disregard for human life. **18.** However, building self-esteem and fighting to love oneself are a part of the culture today in the United States. **19.** Americans may decide that low self-esteem is not a terrible problem, or they may continue to convince themselves that they are good people. **20.** Whatever happens, people today are beginning to debate the value of the idea of self-worth.

◆ 11.1   Run-Ons and Comma Splices

Suggested answers: (Other correct answers are possible.) **1.** The chess-playing computer defeats every student, yet the programmers insist that the machine cannot really think. **2.** Correct **3.** I wanted to wear something else for the photograph; however, I discovered that my favorite outfit no longer fits. **4.** The long-distance telephone company claimed that the problem was with the local one, and the local telephone company blamed the long-distance one. **5.** A regular mole check should be part of an annual physical exam, and any change in a mole should be reported to a doctor immediately. **6.** Correct **7.** The children at the door are collecting for UNICEF. What shall we give them? **8.** Flying is cheaper than taking the train, and on most trips, it also takes less time. **9.** I like compact fluorescent light bulbs because they save energy, but my mother likes them because they do not get hot. **10.** Maria had never realized how violent some fairy tales could be until her daughter had a nightmare after hearing the story of Hansel and Gretel. **11.** No rain had fallen for weeks in the county; nevertheless, the local golf course broke the law by watering the grass. **12.** The toys were antiques that had belonged to Conrad's grandfather, so his mother would not let him touch them. **13.** You should avoid that professor. His tests have nothing to do with the readings he assigns for the class. **14.** My roommate borrowed my sweater, but before she returned it, she had it cleaned. **15.** The song that he had not heard in years brought back a rush of happy childhood memories. **16.** As Jorge floated on his back in the lake, he admired the puffy clouds high in the sky above. **17.** The grammar checker on this computer gives strange advice, so I do not usually use it. **18.** In the poems, Mehitabel is a cat; Archy is a cockroach who was a writer in his previous life. **19.** Jan has not unpacked the boxes in his basement since he moved five years ago; therefore, he probably doesn't really need the items in them. **20.** Correct

♦ **11.2   Run-Ons and Comma Splices**

Answers: Run-ons/comma splices: 2, 3, 5, 7, 8, 9, 10, 12, 14, 15, 16, 17, 18, 20
Suggested answers: (Other correct answers are possible.) **1.** When Americans planted trees in their cities and towns, they often planted American elms. **2.** These trees are tall, and their branches are long and graceful. **3.** Elms look beautiful along a street; the branches on one side form an arch with the branches on the other side. **4.** Settlers put rows and rows of elms along roads to form leafy green avenues. **5.** The elm was one of the most common trees in the United States; in fact, in some towns it was nearly the only type of tree. **6.** Almost every American town has an Elm Street that was named for the stately American elm.

7. Scientists have a name for a landscape with only one type of plant. They call it a monoculture. **8.** Monocultures can cause problems; for example, they are much more likely to suffer an epidemic of a disease. **9.** That is exactly what happened in the case of the American elm. Deadly Dutch elm disease arrived from abroad. **10.** The trees had no resistance to Dutch elm disease, which had no natural enemies in the United States. **11.** The climate where elms grew in the United States was perfect for Dutch elm disease as well. **12.** The disease killed the elm trees across the United States, and in the northern part of the country more than half of all the elms died. **13.** Dutch elm disease can move through the root system from tree to tree when several elms are planted in a row, so the popularity of American elms made the disease worse. **14.** Isolated trees can sometimes be saved. However, that is an expensive and difficult job. **15.** Tree experts find it nearly impossible to save large numbers of elms; instead, they can only look for replacements for the dying trees.

16. American towns today are more likely than in the past to have different kinds of trees and shrubs, for monocultures are not as favored now. **17.** One reason for this change was the total devastation caused by Dutch elm disease. No one wanted that to happen again. **18.** The most susceptible elm trees have already died, but this does not mean that tree diseases from abroad no longer concern Americans. **19.** Dogwoods, oaks, cedars, and redwoods are suffering now from diseases that were unknown in the United States a few decades ago. **20.** Scientists wonder how American trees will respond to such threats, and everyone hopes that no other native species will be hurt as badly as the American elms have been.

♦ **12.1   Sentence Fragments**

Answers: Fragments: 2, 4, 5, 7, 10, 12, 14, 15, 17, 19, 21
Suggested answers: (Other correct answers are possible.) **1.** Michel Nostradame was an astrologer **2.** who lived in the sixteenth century. **3.** Known today as Nostradamus, he wrote four-line poems called quatrains. **4.** A book of these poems was published in 1555 **5.** with the title *Centuries*.

6. These poems were supposed to be prophecies **7.** of events that would happen someday. **8.** The language of the poems was very obscure. **9.** Nevertheless, some people believed that the poems were accurate predictions **10.** and hailed Nostradamus as a man who could see the future.

11. Translations of Nostradamus's poems still sell many copies each year **12.** as new generations hear about the supposed psychic gifts of the sixteenth-century Frenchman. **13.** Skeptical readers notice **14.** that the translations often make the quatrains more specific **15.** to make the predictions clear after the fact. **16.** Some translators change words to add references to people such as Hitler **17.** that do not appear in the original French. **18.** The poems of Nostradamus, carefully translated, are cryptic. **19.** They can be interpreted to mean almost anything. **20.** Psychics today make cryptic predictions that can be claimed to reveal foreknowledge later, **21.** which, as the Nostradamus "prophecies" demonstrates, is a very old trick.

◆ 12.2 Sentence Fragments

Answers: Fragments: 1, 4, 6, 7, 10, 12, 15, 16, 18, 19, 20
Suggested answers: (Other correct answers are possible.) **1.** According to linguistic experts, **2.** Yiddish began in the tenth century, when Jews from northern France settled in towns on the Rhine. **3.** They began to speak the local German dialect **4.** because many medieval Jews did not want to use their sacred language, Hebrew, at home. **5.** However, they wrote the German dialect using Hebrew characters, **6.** avoiding the Roman alphabet because they associated it with Latin, **7.** the language that reminded them of Christian persecution. **8.** Thus, Yiddish became a language of Jewish households and markets in central Europe.

9. Laws in Europe in the twelfth and thirteenth centuries prevented Jews from living near Christians, **10.** leading to the creation of Jewish ghettos. **11.** The segregation of Jews and Christians created language differences between German and Yiddish. **12.** Although Yiddish is officially categorized as Judeo-German, **13.** it has somewhat different spelling and grammar from German. **14.** Yiddish was the most-used language among European Jews until World War II, **15.** when many Yiddish speakers were killed in the Holocaust.

16. With the arrival of many Jews in the United States between the late 1800s and the 1940s, **17.** Yiddish continued to grow **18.** by adding English words. **19.** English, which has borrowed from languages all over the world, **20.** took words, phrases, and other linguistic devices from Yiddish, so both languages were broadened by the exchange.

◆ 13.1 Subject-Verb Agreement

Answers: **1.** has **2.** are **3.** attract **4.** wants **5.** expect **6.** are **7.** looks **8.** come **9.** do **10.** keeps **11.** has **12.** are **13.** Is **14.** do **15.** does **16.** have **17.** takes **18.** deserves **19.** is **20.** have

◆ 13.2 Subject-Verb Agreement

Answers: **1.** do **2.** Correct **3.** charge **4.** wants **5.** Correct; weighs **6.** appears; runs **7.** wear **8.** Correct **9.** do; are **10.** is **11.** have; correct **12.** sounds **13.** needs; does **14.** stop **15.** Correct; correct **16.** frightens

◆ 14.1 Illogical Shifts

Answers: (Other correct answers are possible.) **1.** My father loved this hat, so I have always treasured it. **2.** The rainstorm passed, and by morning a gorgeous sunrise appeared over the mountain. **3.** Many people like the convenience of online shopping, but they have to pay shipping charges. **4.** Correct **5.** Most people watch a lot of television, but few of them want to admit it. **6.** The little girls wanted pink ballerina tutus, but their mother did not like those dresses. **7.** Correct **8.** Correct **9.** We rowed out into the lake and baited our hooks, and in an instant, a big fish struck. **10.** To get a good grade, students should always prepare for exams, and they must keep up with the coursework. **11.** Before you drink the water, you should boil it for twenty minutes. **12.** She is allergic to shellfish, so she did not eat the shrimp. **13.** My grandfather told me to expect a surprise in the mail, and then a fruitcake arrived. **14.** The office staff had to make the coffee, and the workers clearly resented the task. **15.** Correct **16.** Correct **17.** Local youth groups took the newspapers to the recycling center, and the kids also collected cans and glass bottles. **18.** If you want change in the political system, you have to vote. **19.** I was just about to discover the meaning of life, and then I woke up. **20.** Fawzia told her that she could get organic vegetables at the supermarket.

◆ 14.2 Illogical Shifts

Answers: Items containing illogical shifts: 1, 2, 3, 4, 5, 8, 9, 10, 12, 13, 14, 16, 17, 19, 20
Suggested answers: (Other correct answers are possible.) **1.** My friend Angel told me that I could sign up for a bicycle ride across the state. **2.** I had always enjoyed cycling, although I had never ridden such a long distance. **3.** Angel also mentioned that I could get sponsors to agree to pay a certain amount to a charity for every mile cycled. **4.** I decided that I wanted to raise money for a good cause. **5.** I agreed to join the bicycle ride, and I immediately began training. **6.** I wanted to be in good shape for the ride, so I tried to get fit through hard work and practice.

7. For several weeks, I biked twenty or thirty miles each day. **8.** By late spring, when the statewide ride was scheduled to begin, I felt ready to go. **9.** I had found sponsors to contribute to the charity, and all I had to do now was pedal five hundred miles. **10.** Angel had planned to ride, too, but he injured his knee in March. **11.** I asked his sponsors if they would sponsor me instead, and most agreed. **12.** With the potential to earn so much for a good cause, I suddenly realized how important it was for me to complete the ride. **13.** Angel told me that I shouldn't think about things like that before a long, strenuous trip.

14. We set out on our bikes in May, riding from west to east so that we would not be facing into the wind. **15.** The western half of the state has higher hills and elevations, so we could also make better time by traveling east. **16.** We wanted to do the hardest part of the trip at the beginning, when we were fresh. **17.** On the first day, fast-moving trucks passed us, and the weather was rainy and miserable. **18.** However, I never really thought about quitting because I couldn't have faced the sponsors and the people at the charity if I had quit. **19.** To my surprise, I soon found that I was one of the strongest and fastest cyclists in the group. **20.** I completed the five-hundred-mile trip a day ahead of schedule, and the charity received a large contribution.

◆ 15.1 Dangling and Misplaced Modifiers

Suggested answers: (Other correct answers are possible.) **1.** Sweating in the humid sunshine, the workers drove the tractors back and forth across the field. **2.** Certain of danger, the beaver smacked the water with its broad tail. **3.** Exhausted after the long drive, we pulled our car into the driveway at last. **4.** Water kept dripping out of the vase handmade by my niece. **5.** That book that I borrowed from you kept me awake far into the night. **6.** A reflecting pool filled with carp surrounded the temple. **7.** With nowhere else to turn, she decided that the bus station was her only option. **8.** Pretending to smile, dancing contestants covered the stage. **9.** The weather turned suddenly cold, and snow began to fall. **10.** She used paste made of flour and water to put the flowers in the book. **11.** The letter carrier tiptoed around the dog snarling defiantly. **12.** Aching from the long hike, my foot got a huge blister from a hole in my sock. **13.** Taping the bow on top, I thought the package looked perfect. **14.** Stuck in the ditch, I had never found the mobile phone more useful. **15.** The dead tree with a hole in it attracted a squirrel family. **16.** We discovered an ancient type of beetle preserved in amber. **17.** Gothic novels featuring old castles and mysterious strangers thrill many readers. **18.** Hundreds of feet over our heads, the blimp floated past, making us gasp. **19.** I accidentally sent an e-mail intended for you alone to the whole class. **20.** Stunned by the revelation, the people in the banquet hall made no sound.

◆ 15.2 Dangling and Misplaced Modifiers

Answers: Items containing dangling and misplaced modifiers: 1, 2, 3, 4, 5, 6, 8, 9, 10, 11, 12, 13, 15, 16, 17, 18, 19

Suggested answers: (Other correct answers are possible.) **1.** An abandoned house filled with cobwebs and mysterious rooms attracted three neighborhood children. **2.** Creeping in through the broken window by the porch, they saw that nothing had been disturbed for decades. **3.** A calendar on the wall said that the date was October 1977. **4.** Looking first in the kitchen, Sam, Dana, and Eduardo were surprised to find the cupboards filled with boxes and cans. **5.** Eduardo picked up a can of beans with an ancient yellow label. **6.** The children saw that mice scuttling across the floor had made the house their own. **7.** Boxes of cereal with contents that had long ago been eaten by rodents remained on the shelves.

8. Inching up the steps, the children thought the creaks and groans sounded human. **9.** The house that had been empty for so long seemed to be speaking to the children. **10.** The furnishings, covered with a thick layer of dust, reminded them of things they had seen at their grandparents' houses. **11.** Sam, the oldest of the three, wanted to look in the attic. **12.** Climbing up the ladder to the top of the house, they discovered treasures. **13.** Old clothes from the disco era spilled out of a battered suitcase. **14.** Dana put on a glittery shirt with sequins that spelled out "Boogie." **15.** Eduardo tried a pair of platform shoes with four-inch wooden heels.

16. Returning to the house a week later, the three children brought along a portable CD player. **17.** Sam, Dana, and Eduardo, unable to stop giggling, opened the suitcase. **18.** Sam played a copy of *ABBA's Greatest Hits* borrowed from his mother's collection. **19.** The three, adorned with shoes, hats, giant sunglasses, and yards of polyester, danced through the attic. **20.** Echoing with laughter, the old house seemed to welcome the children's lively presence.

◆ 16.1 Verbs: Past Tense

Answers: **1.** decided **2.** crossed **3.** skied **4.** covered **5.** pulled **6.** appeared (arrived) **7.** awarded **8.** honored **9.** saved **10.** searched **11.** collapsed **12.** helped **13.** arrived (appeared) **14.** burned **15.** brushed **16.** worked **17.** walked **18.** scorched **19.** mailed **20.** contributed

◆ 16.2 Verbs: Past Tense

Answers: **1.** began **2.** started **3.** saw **4.** did **5.** published **6.** sold **7.** sent **8.** gave **9.** took **10.** became **11.** grew **12.** was **13.** worked **14.** reached **15.** graduated **16.** studied **17.** taught **18.** took **19.** had **20.** founded

◆ 17.1 Verbs: Past Participles

Answers: **1.** known; hidden **2.** broken; beaten **3.** slept; awoken **4.** thrown; caught **5.** written; thought; torn **6.** spoken; seen **7.** worn **8.** eaten; grown **9.** dived; swum **10.** paid; spent **11.** has sworn **12.** had taught **13.** had boiled **14.** has felt **15.** had raised **16.** had left **17.** have met **18.** has written **19.** had spent **20.** had frozen

◆ 17.2 Verbs: Past Participles

Answers: **1.** correct, correct **2.** had lighted (had lit) **3.** had patented, correct **4.** correct, had joined **5.** had been, correct **6.** had taken **7.** have relied **8.** correct **9.** has made **10.** have wondered, correct **11.** have gone **12.** have kept **13.** correct, used **14.** has emerged **15.** correct

◆ 18.1 Nouns

Answers: **1.** cardiologists **2.** Federation **3.** organization; Geneva, Switzerland **4.** spokesman; depression **5.** emotions, person's **6.** husbands-to-be; wives-to-be **7.** Professor; Poole-Wilson; Imperial College **8.** dishes; potatoes **9.** scientists **10.** proofs; beliefs **11.** study; men; women; coronary **12.** Half; patients; lives **13.** participants; relationship **14.** children **15.** ponies **16.** zoo; friends **17.** wishes **18.** These; people

◆ 18.2 Nouns

Answers: **1.** people **2.** correct, populations **3.** monkeys **4.** groups, mice, correct **5.** models **6.** correct **7.** deer, elk **8.** Critics **9.** correct **10.** Wolves **11.** Grizzlies **12.** correct, dolphins, mammals **13.** correct, fishermen **14.** fish **15.** geese **16.** correct, sanctuaries, correct **17.** correct

◆ 19.1 Pronouns

Answers: **1.** I **2.** it **3.** He **4.** his or her **5.** its **6.** themselves **7.** He and she **8.** its **9.** We **10.** his or her **11.** their **12.** his or her **13.** him; me **14.** they; their **15.** I **16.** his **17.** We **18.** me **19.** me **20.** him; her

◆ 19.2 Pronouns

Answers: Everyone is aware of the importance of exercise in maintaining *his or her* health. School children exercise *themselves* once they are let loose in the schoolyard at recess. Many older children become involved in organized sports, so that team workouts and games become *their* exercise program. And, of course, *we* adults fill gyms and fitness centers to keep our bodies strong and fit.

However, exercise for babies, toddlers, and preschoolers is often ignored. Parents assume they get enough exercise by *themselves*. When a parent or caretaker is busy, *he or she* may keep a baby or toddler confined in *his or her* stroller, baby seat, or play pen for too long. But, every young child needs exercise, or *he or she* may not develop at a normal rate. *Experts* recommend that caregivers involve even very young children in fun physical activities in order to keep *them* healthy.

My wife and *I* have spent time exercising our daughter Erin since she was a baby. Because Erin spent time on a blanket on the floor instead of in a play pen or bouncy seat, the baby got a lot of practice rolling *herself* over. Erin and I played endless games of "pattycake" and "peekaboo." When Erin was a toddler, *experts (our doctor)* told us that toddlers should have at least 30 minutes of physical activity spread throughout the day. During these play periods, we got *her* to move along with a song or play ball with *us*. I threw soft balls that *she* caught and threw back. Now Erin is a 9-year-old who can pitch for *her* baseball team. Our doctor also recommended that Erin have "free play" time for *her* to explore, push, and pull objects as well as balancing and climbing on safe surfaces. All this hard work has given *us* a healthy, energetic child.

◆ 20.1 Adjectives and Adverbs

Answers: **1.** funniest **2.** well; well **3.** wisest **4.** better **5.** best **6.** really; directly **7.** bad; badly **8.** fully **9.** worse **10.** easier **11.** This; that **12.** more strongly **13.** quickly **14.** well; better **15.** healthier; more dangerous **16.** this; that **17.** worse; worst **18.** good; well **19.** this; that **20.** well; good

◆ 20.2 Adjectives and Adverbs

Answers: **1.** The sport of ice climbing has become *really* popular in recent years. **2.** Most ice climbers try this sport after mastering rock climbing, which is the *easier* of the two. **3.** Climbing an icy slope is *more dangerous* than climbing a mountain in *warmer* weather. **4.** In order to do *well* at ice climbing, you need to first gain experience climbing *more solid* rocks.

5. Enthusiasts say that they love the physical and mental challenge of climbing in freezing and often wet weather on more *slippery surfaces*. **6.** Many say the ice is *more beautiful* than anything they have ever seen. **7.** Some say they like being *more scared* than they have ever been too. **8.** Ice climbers progress from climbing mountain slopes of 45 degrees to *more challenging* frozen waterfalls that are almost vertical sheets of ice.

9. However, the sport has become *safer* in recent years. **10.** This is the result of *better* equipment and climbing techniques. **11.** Climbers wear plastic or insulated leather boots with crampons attached to the bottom. **12.** These crampons have 10 or 12 metal "teeth" that help feet grip the ice *more tightly*. **13.** In a technique called "top-roping," a metal connector is planted *securely* at the top of the climbing surface, and a rope is hung from it. **14.** This feat is done by the *most experienced* climber in the group. **15.** *This* climber makes his or her way up the ice by driving an axe or pick into the ice. **16.** Climbers use their boots and crampons to gain footholds in the ice. **17.** These actions are made safer because climbers wear harnesses that are attached to the rope held in place by the connector at the top. **18.** The best ice climbers use *deliberate* moves to climb *efficiently* up the ice. **19.** Beginners are usually *more wasteful* of their energy. **20.** They climb too *forcefully* and get tired too *quickly*.

◆ 21.1 Grammar and Usage Issues for ESL Writers

Answers: **1.** It wasn't a good idea. **2.** She learned to play golf so she could join her husband on weekends. **3.** My brother went back to Afghanistan to teach school. **4.** When a rap song blasted on the radio, the song woke Hiroshi from a deep sleep. **5.** The worst experience I ever had was that I was separated from my family for a year and didn't know where they were. **6.** The children brought a lot of sand into the house from the beach outside. **7.** I received ten pieces of mail today. **8.** Margit drinks her tea with two sugars and a little milk. **9.** There are many obstacles to finding a suitable place to live. **10.** If there are chocolate cookies around, I can't eat one cookie and stop there. **11.** Most people need routine as well as stimulation in their lives. **12.** Siri and her family live on Montgomery Street near the East Side Highway. **13.** Our school library has many computers available to students. **14.** Both red-haired twin boys have freckled faces. **15.** Please don't worry about that problem. **16.** Who is teaching the class tomorrow? **17.** The engine needs some oil or it won't run well. **18.** That ugly, broken-down, orange reclining chair should be thrown out. **19.** The charity was grateful for our large donation. **20.** Our lawyer objected to the judge's decision.

◆ 21.2 Grammar and Usage Issues for ESL Writers

Answers: **1.** Last year, I moved from my noisy city neighborhood to a small house on a quiet country road. **2.** I knew my new life would contrast with my old one. **3.** I didn't realize how different it would be. **4.** At first, the quiet of the country bothered me. **5.** The first night I was in my new home, I heard strange noises outside. **6.** There were loud noises like singing all night. **7.** The next day, I learned that these noises were made by many tiny frogs called "peepers."
    8. In my city apartment building, I didn't have much contact with my neighbors. **9.** But, on my country road, my next-door neighbors made sure that I became acquainted with them. **10.** They invited me for coffee and pie. **11.** I was grateful for their friendliness. **12.** In fact, now we are good friends. **13.** We depend on each other for small favors, like watching each other's pets when we are away.
    14. Life in my small country town differs from city life in many ways. **15.** I can take advantage of many outdoor activities. **16.** Many months of the year, I am busy in my garden. **17.** There are many places to swim, hike, climb mountains, and ride a bicycle. **18.** I am also pleased with the spirit in my home town. **19.** Everyone works together to protect nature against destruction. **20.** When my city friends ask me if I'm bored with living in a small country town, I reply, "No way!"

◆ 22.1 Using Commas

Answers: **1.** Joan Kroc, widow of the founder of McDonald's hamburger restaurants, gives generously to many causes. **2.** In fact, she is one of the top philanthropists in America. **3.** She has contributed over $150 million dollars to help the disadvantaged, heal the sick, house the homeless, and promote world peace. **4.** In 1982, the year her husband died, Mrs. Kroc founded Ronald McDonald House Charities. **5.** Named after the famous clown, Ronald McDonald Houses are residences near hospitals where families of seriously ill children can stay. **6.** Over the years, Joan Kroc has donated more than $100 million dollars to this foundation. **7.** Today, the organization sponsors children's health charities in 32 countries. **8.** Much of her giving, however, is closer to home. **9.** Mrs. Kroc is a resident of San Diego, California. **10.** After witnessing the poverty in southeast San Diego, Joan Kroc donated 80 million dollars to the Salvation Army to build a community center there. **11.** Currently, the center provides local children with before- and after-school programs in academic subjects, sports, and creative and performing arts, such as music, acting, art, and dancing. **12.** The center, a large complex, includes a gymnasium, a 500-seat theater, a library filled with computers, a swimming pool, an ice skating rink, and facilities for a variety of sports. **13.** Correct **14.** In addition, Mrs. Kroc has donated money to help flood victims in Grand Forks, North Dakota, to AIDS research, and to rehabilitation programs. **15.** Recently, Joan Kroc has focused her giving on the issue of world peace. **16.** She donated 6 million dollars to the University of Notre Dame to establish an Institute for International Peace Studies where, hopefully, workable plans for world peace can be created. **17.** A few years later, she founded the Kroc Institute for Peace and Justice at the University of San Diego. **18.** At the Institute, political leaders, scholars, students, and activists gather to work together in the cause of peace. **19.** In response to the attacks of September 11, 2001, both institutes are busier than ever. **20.** Joan Kroc, a person who cares about peace, is making a contribution toward a better future for everyone.

◆ 22.2   Using Commas

Answers: **1.** To scientists, a fossil is not just the remains of a long-dead plant or animal. **2.** The name *trace fossil* can be given to any evidence that living creatures were once in a particular area. **3.** For example, dinosaur footprints are just as much fossils as dinosaur bones and teeth. **4.** Worms burrowed through soil millions of years ago, claim experts. **5.** Tunnels in the soil, now hardened into rock, reveal what the worms were like. **6.** Molds, another type of trace fossil, are formed when bones, shells, and other hard materials make an imprint in mud. **7.** These molds show what the animal or plant looked like, even without remains.

8. Fossils are most often found in layers of rock that were formed from sand, mud, shells, and other materials. **9.** Over thousands of years, water washes over buried objects like bones, teeth, and shells in the ground. **10.** Minerals from the water gradually replace all or part of the object, creating a hard fossil. **11.** As time goes by, that fossil becomes embedded in the rock.

12. Paleontologists, scientists who study ancient forms of life, get a lot of information from fossils. **13.** For instance, they can figure out from an animal's footprint how tall it was, how much it weighed, and how it moved around. **14.** Animal droppings can tell what the creature ate. **15.** The most revealing fossils are bodies of animals that have dried out in the desert or were preserved in ice or tar. **16.** For this reason, we know what woolly mammoths, shaggy elephant-like beasts from over a million years ago, looked like. **17.** The La Brea tar pits in Los Angeles, California, became a burial place for many Ice Age animals. **18.** The bones of saber-toothed tigers, giant ground sloths, and mammoths have all been found in the tar pits. **19.** The George C. Page Museum, right near the tar pits, contains skeletons of these animals. **20.** Since 1906, scientists have been studying these remains.

◆ 23.1   Using Apostrophes

Answers: **1.** The New York City firefighters' bravery brought them national recognition. **2.** You won't believe the story I just heard. **3.** Everyone says that's not what happened. **4.** Their apartment is identical in size and layout to ours. **5.** Correct **6.** Women's fashions can change drastically from year to year, while men's remain pretty much the same. **7.** Who's in charge of payroll at this company? **8.** The girls carefully stored their hockey equipment after the game. **9.** Correct **10.** The Riveras' house is right next door to theirs. **11.** The school board gave all the principals a raise. **12.** Let's find out if this lost handbag is hers. **13.** Correct **14.** Wouldn't it be better to buy those sneakers on sale? **15.** John Adams's son, John Quincy Adams, was this country's sixth president. **16.** A knight's suit of armor protected the warrior's entire body. **17.** Sandra Cisneros's stories of Hispanic life always touch my heart. **18.** It's fun to watch the kitten play with its toy. **19.** If everybody tried to understand the beliefs of others, we'd all get along better. **20.** The business's profits have gone up but its stock has not done the same.

◆ 23.2   Using Apostrophes

Answers: **1.** Many people's reaction to a dentist's chair is one of fear. **2.** One dentist estimates that over 90 percent of her patients are fearful of dental work. **3.** "Sometimes they'll get nervous just hearing the drill," she says, "even when the teeth being drilled aren't theirs. **4.** . . . I've been bitten a lot, too, and most of the time it's an accident," she asserts. **5.** But she also suspects that a few bites have been on purpose. **6.** Because this dentist is a wholesome-looking young woman, patients have told her, "You don't look like someone who'd be a dentist." **7.** It's even worse when they find out that she's a specialist in root canals.

8. Our teeth's tendency to decay has caused painful problems for millions of years. **9.** In pre-historic times, there wasn't much to do but pull out a rotted tooth. **10.** Later, wealthy Egyptians, Greeks, and Romans of ancient times could replace their teeth with fake gold ones. **11.** The jeweler's skill was employed to make false teeth in the Middle Ages. **12.** However, pulling teeth was usually the barber's job. **13.** Later, surgeons took over. **14.** A French dental scientist, Pierre Fauchard, published a treatise called *The Surgeon Dentist* in 1728. **15.** The book's illustrations showed dental tools and devices of the time. **16.** In 1840, the world's first dental school opened its doors in Baltimore, Maryland. **17.** Here's what a visit to the dentist's office would have been like around 1850. **18.** Ether or nitrous oxide would've been used to make you unconscious before painful procedures. **19.** Now there are local anesthetics that block pain only in the area the dentist is working on. **20.** Let's all be thankful for the advances that minimize pain in modern dentistry.

◆ 24.1   Understanding Mechanics

Answers: **1.** "I am still skeptical about this new discovery," said the scientist from Princeton University. **2.** Joelle's math class meets Tuesday afternoon in Olin Hall. **3.** Jerry Seinfeld was a popular comedian even before he starred in the television series *Seinfeld*. **4.** Many Muslims make a pilgrimage to Mecca in Saudi Arabia as part of their religious practice. **5.** The writer Annie Dillard said, "The secret of seeing is to sail on solar wind." **6.** Some of the Chinese-American characters in Amy Tan's book *The Joy Luck Club* live on Sacramento Street. **7.** My brother Louis, who joined the Boy Scouts in February, said that he looks forward to hiking and camping at the lake near our town. **8.** In his poem "The Waste Land," T. S. Eliot wrote, "April is the cruelest month." **9.** A story in *Time* magazine praised Denzel Washington's performance as a civil rights leader in the movie *Malcolm X*. **10.** The computer company Microsoft, which developed the program Microsoft Explorer, is located east of Seattle in Redmond, Washington. **11.** In History 111, we studied the Revolutionary War and the United States Constitution. **12.** The Jewish holiday of Passover, which takes place in the spring, includes many special foods. **13.** You may know that Uncle Robert, who can speak both English and French, is fond of saying, "Speaking two languages is like having two minds." **14.** The Department of Environmental Conservation is responsible for protecting natural resources such as rivers and forests. **15.** In *The Wizard of Oz*, Dorothy clicks her heels together and says, "There's no place like home." **16.** Like many who held the office before him, President George W. Bush was once a state governor. **17.** The Centerville Garden Club meets the first Tuesday of every month except in winter. **18.** "If we are going to be the next Ford Motor Company," said the manager, "employees will have to be here on time Monday morning." **19.** The Americans and the Japanese fought some of the Second World War's fiercest battles on islands in the Pacific Ocean. **20.** Correct

◆ 24.2   Understanding Mechanics

Answers: **1.** There is a long tradition of travel in the United States. **2.** For one thing, the nation is made up of people from other places, including Europe, Africa, and Asia. **3.** The earliest settlers landed on the shores of what are now Massachusetts and Virginia. **4.** It did not take long for the mostly English settlers to found cities such as Boston and Philadelphia. **5.** They also built Harvard University, which was originally a Christian college.

6. Throughout their history, Americans have been restless. **7.** "Go west, young man," is a famous quotation from the nation's pioneer days. **8.** People crossed the Mississippi River in great numbers to establish farms and businesses. **9.** They encountered driving snow in January and February and intense heat in summer. **10.** Still, many succeeded in reaching the West.

11. Today, people travel to see the country and its best known places, including the Statue of Liberty in New York City and Bourbon Street in New Orleans. **12.** The American Association for Retired Persons and similar groups organize trips and tours. **13.** The *New York Times* and other newspapers have travel sections, with articles such as "Finding the Best Hotel in Minneapolis." **14.** The week after Christmas is an especially popular time to travel, when people visit Uncle Bob and Aunt Sue or go skiing in the Rocky Mountains. **15.** "The winter is the best time to travel," one travel agent said, "because most people need a change at that time of year."

16. Many stories have been written about travel, including Jack Kerouac's book *On the Road*. **17.** Woody Guthrie wrote a famous song about places in the United States. **18.** In it, he sang, "This land was made for you and me." **19.** That statement is still true today, as people travel from the Pacific Ocean to the Atlantic Ocean, perhaps hearing Spanish spoken in Houston and Chinese in Chicago. **20.** No class in history or geography could be as rewarding as seeing America's deserts, rivers, mountains, and people firsthand.

◆ 25.1 Understanding Spelling

Answers: **1.** piece, roommate **2.** restaurant, beginning **3.** everyone, correct, careful **4.** overrates, acting **5.** correct, senseless **6.** relief, correct **7.** correct, embarrassed, tries **8.** dryness, digging **9.** correct, a lot, insurance **10.** spied, correct, government **11.** surprised, correct, excelled, writing **12.** ceiling, entrance, correct **13.** women, correct, potato **14.** correct, playful **15.** argument, Wednesday **16.** correct, dissatisfied **17.** friend, probably, runners **18.** grammar, creating, correct, interesting **19.** occurred, correct **20.** generally, correct, answered, scientists

◆ 25.2 Understanding Spelling

Answers: **1.** Change *certian* to *certain* **2.** Change *definate* to *definite* **3.** Change *nowing* to *knowing* **4.** Change *erly* to *early* **5.** Change *anceint* to *ancient*; *dependant* to *dependent*; *livelyhood* to *livelihood* **6.** Change *noticable* to *noticeable*; *occured* to *occurred* **7.** Change *truely* to *truly*; *calender* to *calendar* **8.** Change *placment* to *placement* **9.** Change *begining* to *beginning* **10.** Change *displaied* to *displayed* **11.** Change *climed* to *climbed* **12.** Change *minuet* to *minute*; *untill* to *until* **13.** Change *judgement* to *judgment*; *planing* to *planning* **14.** Change *tinyer* to *tinier* **15.** Change *Finaly* to *Finally*; *fourty* to *forty* **16.** Change *happenning* to *happening* **17.** Change *destroied* to *destroyed*; *liesurely* to *leisurely* **18.** Change *beleive* to *believe* **19.** Change *simpley* to *simply* **20.** Change *enjoiment* to *enjoyment*

◆ 26.1 Learning Commonly Confused Words

Answers: **1.** accepted, quite **2.** hear, correct, they're **3.** loose, effect **4.** correct, plain, it's **5.** principal, sit, quietly **6.** by, correct, where **7.** supposed, except **8.** conscious, mind **9.** correct, then, brake **10.** threw, correct, than **11.** here, already, correct **12.** correct, lie, no **13.** breaking **14.** knew, buy, two **15.** all ready, correct **16.** find, correct **17.** passed, conscience **18.** lies, every day **19.** your, correct, too **20.** past, used, correct

◆ 26.2 Learning Commonly Confused Words

Answers: **1.** Change *too* to *to* **2.** Change *sit* to *set*; *every day* to *everyday* **3.** Change *fine* to *find*; *quite* to *quiet* **4.** Change *by* to *buy* **5.** Change *suppose* to *supposed*; *use* to *used* **6.** Change *whose* to *who's*; *plane* to *plain* **7.** Change *affects* to *effects*; *know* to *no* **8.** Change *than* to *then*; *here* to *hear* **9.** Change *principle* to *principal* **10.** Change *passed* to *past*; *rise* to *raise* **11.** Change *find* to *fine* **12.** Change *set* to *sit*; *lose* to *loose* **13.** Change *through* to *threw*; *were* to *where*; *write* to *right* **14.** Change *they're* to *their* **15.** Change *pieceful* to *peaceful* **16.** Change *its* to *it's*